LABORATORY

Quality Systems | Quality Assurance
Standardization | Accreditation

Quality Management

MANUAL

The Authors

Pamposh Kumar

is a scientist with the Department of Science and Technology, Goverment of India (GOI), New Delhi. An organic chemist, he has had wide experience at the National Board for Testing and Calibration Laboratories (NABL), especially as convener for accreditation of clinical and photomatry testing laboratories, and with the documentation for the NABL accreditation system. He was involved in drawing up the technical criteria for these fields (including forensic and DNA fingerprinting laboratories) of testing for accreditation at NABL. He also has a long experience in coordination and management of sponsored Research and Technology Development. Prior to this he was a researcher at the National Institute of Immunology, New Delhi. He is a life member of Materials Research Society of India (MRSI).

V.P.S. Tomar

is a scientist with the Department of Science and Technology, Ministry of Science and Technology, GOI, New Delhi. A mechanical engineer by qualification, he has had a long stint at the National Board for Testing and Calibration Laboratories (NABL), New Delhi. He has been involved with mechanical testing laboratories, as convener with accreditation of chemical testing laboratories, and also the documentation for the NABL accreditation system. Previously he held senior positions in the area of quality assurance/quality control at Bureau of Indian Standards and Tehri-Hydro Development Corporation Limited. Besides having rich experience of coordinating and managing Research and Technology Development at DST, he has been a professional mechanical engineer at various private firms. He also holds a degree in law.

LABORATORY

Quality Systems | Quality Assurance
Standardization | Accreditation
Quality Management

MANUAL

Pamposh Kumar • V.P.S. Tomar

CBS

CBS PUBLISHERS & DISTRIBUTORS

NEW DELHI • BANGALORE

LABORATORY
Quality Systems
Quality Assurance
Standardisation
Accreditation
Quality Management
MANUAL

ISBN : 81-239-1231-5

First Edition: 2005

Production Director : Vinod K. Jain

Published by :
Satish Kumar Jain for CBS Publishers & Distributors,
4596/1-A, 11 Darya Ganj, New Delhi - 110 002 (India)
E-mail : cbspubs@vsnl.com
Website : www.cbspd.com

Branch Office :
Seema House, 2975, 17th Cross, K.R. Road,
Bansankari 2nd Stage, Bangalore - 560070
Fax : 080-6771680 • E-mail : cbsbng@vsnl.net

Typeset at : CBS Publishers & Distributors, Typesetting unit

Printed at : S.D.R. Printers Delhi-94

to

our

parents

Foreword

While the quality movements in almost every sphere of business have the advantage of good books to support meeting the standards, in the field of laboratory accreditation, particularly with the advent of stringent ISO 17025 standard, there is an alarming dearth of user-friendly publications. This book, being the first of its kind at national and international level, is unique in many respects — in terms of clarity and content, in terms of pragmatic and thorough exposition of the subject matter, etc. It deals with all the integral components of preparing for, developing and standardizing the laboratory procedures and quality systems in accordance with the requirements of ISO 17025: 1999, which is fundamental to understanding the challenges in seeking accreditation from any national or international accreditation body. Most of the laboratory managers are unacquainted with these nuances and practical necessities, and therefore may be compelled to hire consultancy services for the work involved. It is not desirable and also sometimes not feasible to achieve the required level of conformity through a consultant alone. Therefore, acquiring the skills of designing, developing, documenting and maintaining the competency required under terms of accreditation is imperative for the laboratory managers, laboratory quality executives, personnel, students and other quality management professionals including teachers at technical and management institutions dealing with the subject. The lapses arising due to lack of a handy knowledge in this area may have serious attendant cost implications, not to speak of a fall in credibility of the laboratory. To overcome this handicap, the authors have brought out in this invaluable book the step-by-step procedures from the start-up stage.

I am delighted to note that the authors have dealt with the most difficult part of the task, preparing the Quality Manual, by giving a lucid account of the issues involved, in do-it-yourself format. This innovative book, drawn on the practical and rich experience of the authors in dealing with laboratories going through the accreditation process, also carries a template of the Quality Manual which, I am sure, shall make the task of acquiring accreditation extraordinarily simple. Very commendably, the authors and the publishers have produced a delectable and exceedingly useful publication, which shall go a long way in helping us respond with standardization of laboratory services quality to the demands of this era of globalization of trade and technology.

Dr. Mahesh Chander Gupta

Advisor, Saudi Arabian Standards Organization (SASO),
Riyadh, Saudi Arabia, and formerly
Head, National Calibration Programme (National Accreditation Board for Testing and Calibration Laboratories),
National Physical Laboratory, New Delhi.
President, Association for Quality Assurance.

Acknowledgement

This book is result of constant encouragement and excellent project management by Mr Y.N. Arjuna, Publishing Director, CBS Publishers & Distributors. It is enriched with his remarkable perception of the laboratory services and their users, which is a direct outcome of his experiences spent at the All India Institute of Medical Sciences, New Delhi, which he shared so liberally with us to augment the simplicity and readability to the volume. We are overwhelmed with his faith in the place for quality in technical education, management and businesses. We wish to place on record our acknowledgement of his valuable support to this publication. We also wish to acknowledge the invaluable work on the manuscript by the typesetting unit of CBS Publishers. Special thanks are also due to Director, Shriram Institute for Industrial Research, Delhi, for permitting the use of photographs of their laboratory facilities.

Pamposh Kumar
V.P.S. Tomar

Preface

Test and calibration laboratories are supposed to be efficient systems which can carry out measurements with required degrees of reliability as assured by accepted standards or expressed demands of a particular client. Consequently, it is natural that the customers of an independent test or calibration laboratory generally want to know how reliable their test or calibration results are. The standard way for the laboratories is to show its customer that the laboratory has adopted laboratory accreditation requirements as mentioned in ISO Guide 25:1990 (now ISO/IEC 17025: 1999) known as "General Requirements for Competence of Testing and Calibration Laboratories". These requirements mean up-gradation of the laboratory's quality system and technical operations accordingly.

There are numerous instances when the concerned laboratory has adopted the laboratory accreditation requirements but not been accredited by a national or international accreditation body.

Such laboratories face plenty of difficulties in formulating their quality system documentation which is the backbone of laboratory accreditation. In the process of developing the quality system documentation for the first time the laboratory has to develop a thinking whereupon the laboratory can start its documentation.

As ISO/IEC 17025:1999 (General Requirements for Competence of Testing and Calibration Laboratories) has already superseded the ISO/IEC Guide 25: 1990, the laboratory accreditation requirements of the latest standard will now have to be complied by the applicant laboratories on demands from the national or international accreditation body.

The book is going to be useful also to accredited laboratories which need to update their quality system documentation to meet the requirements of latest standard.

The book is organized in three parts :

Part I : Laboratory Accreditation
Part II : Laboratory Quality System Documentation
Part III : Writing a Laboratory Quality Manual

The first part deals with the elementary ideas about accreditation, and the steps to acquire laboratory accreditation based on ISO/IEC Guide 25 (1990) or ISO/IEC 17025 (1999). The applicability of prevalent financial obligations, co-operation expected on the part of the applicant laboratory or accredited laboratories, and also the technical requirements are covered in this part.

The second part of the book exclusively deals with quality system documentation required for implementation of ISO/IEC Guide 25:1990 or ISO/IEC 17025: 1999. This part takes care that an applicant laboratory while applying to national or international accreditation body should have already developed its quality manual, quality procedures, standard operating procedures and quality records.

> It has been experienced that the laboratories face difficulties in framing their "Laboratory Quality Policy" and its subject matter. The laboratory has to have thoughts while formulating its Laboratory Quality Policy which is the beginning of laboratory quality management. Keeping in view the importance and real difficulties in framing the same, a full chapter is included in the second part of the book and we are sure that it will help laboratories to write laboratory quality policy in a better way.

The third part of the book deals with the most important document, the Laboratory Quality Manual, which is sought first at hand by an accreditation body before proceeding with the case of the applicant laboratory towards accreditation. Attempts have been made to provide step by step guidance for preparation of all kind of laboratory quality system documentation along with appropriate examples for understanding of the applicant laboratories. A "Guiding Sample for Quality Manual" complying with the requirements of ISO/IEC Guide 17025 (1999) has been presented which shall be immensely helpful to laboratories in formulating their own Quality Manuals without much difficulties.

However, the advice to laboratory quality managers is that while preparing for laboratory quality system, the documentation for their test or calibration laboratory must be realistic to its last detail. It must address the general as well as specific requirements as laid down for laboratory accreditation by the concerned accreditation body. All quality documentation should contain realistic and obtainable norms. A highly accurate and credible laboratory quality system shall lead the laboratory to successful and effective implementation of ISO requirements.

This is an attempt to facilitate the quality conscious laboratories (test or calibration) in formulation and implementation of laboratory quality system documentation. We tried our best to make it useful and practicable to the maximum possible extent based upon our little knowledge and experience in such a vast area of laboratory accreditation. We expect that this will be able to achieve its purpose. As anywhere there are chances for further improvements, the same is applicable to this effort. The comments of readers and laboratory managers are welcome for the betterment of the book.

Pamposh Kumar
V.P.S. Tomar

Contents

APPENDICES

Prologue

Quality Assurance and Meeting the Future

Quality generation is a lifetime job. Assuring it to oneself and to one's clients is a whole time affair. It also goes beyond establishing the quality systems, their standardization and accreditation of their conformity to recognized standards or criteria.

Laboratory services are crucial link in the fast changing businesses and life of today. This link has to be renovated keeping pace with the emerging new needs and those lying in the lap of future. Almost all renovations have costs attached with them. However avoiding the costs can be perilous to objectives of surviving, managing and outgrowing the future. Therefore a logical, thorough, well anticipated and planned renovation of existing quality systems, establishment of additional or newer laboratory quality systems and maintaining their conformity to standards needs a blue print of the necessary steps. Such blue prints are stepping stones on this evolutionary journey and serve as means to escape a costly, frustrating future.

This should also result in continuous re-integration of the quality system with the management system in spite of the updated and many quality manuals. For this it is necessary that the quality assurance (QA) specialists do not view their role as verifiers and the quality reviews do not become a trivial matter of acceptance.

Adoption of good quality management practices is part of other tasks as a continuing trend in quality. Professionals in related fields, such as production, design and purchasing, now have to increasingly follow good quality practice as a normal procedure in their professional work. Quality system standards should be addressed as foundational, not as the ultimate in total quality management practice. Further, the major commitments in the organizations' approach to quality now have to advance from best practices to best-value solutions.

The role of new tools like measurement and reporting in real time and maintenance documentation with the help of software now needs to be given increased and proper place. Further, the QA function is not to be like that of enforcement authority, however, it must take note of deviations from organization's standards and the management should rationally decide on short-term needs versus the long-term benefits of the new system.

Employing a "creditable" expert is not the solution to achieve this dynamic efficiency as he may try to impose his personal inclinations upon the management and staff and may even reject a new practice or technique he does not understand. It is also another matter that such devices result in regarding quality assurance as a system of client's evaluation as against internal review. Instead, it is better to utilize the

`Quality Assurance Focus' as a sounding board and point of reference as a means of systemic approach, and as a communication mechanism for personnel with common problems. Effective use may be made of online check lists and the quality assurance toolkits, benchmarking criteria, rating systems and best practices. This shall be helpful in integrating quality assurance procedures into working practices. It has also been demonstrated to beneficially carry out the procedures in key areas of quality assurance like Strategic Quality Assurance (to be carried out before development taking place), Workflow Quality Assurance (to be carried out before and during development), Sign-off Quality Assurance (to be carried out as concluding Quality Assurance, as auditing system after one stage of development is over) and most importantly the On-going Quality Assurance (to be carried out in establishing a system to report, check, and correct any shortcoming found). These key areas, as the basis of over all quality assurance, are highly beneficial for acquiring the current and future quality levels.

While it is true that many organizations have quality assurance at the level of conformance and compliance with specifications and corrective actions and are not working with the prevention-based, proactive quality systems, tomorrow's quality assurance will have to have a focus on being strategy-driven and with a significant emphasis not only on today's customers but also future customers and markets. Therefore, tomorrow's quality revolution would develop systems based on autonomy and freedom, which would in turn allow people to create quality.

EFFICIENT UTILIZATION OF TECHNICAL PERSONNEL, PROCEDURES AND INSTRUMENTS

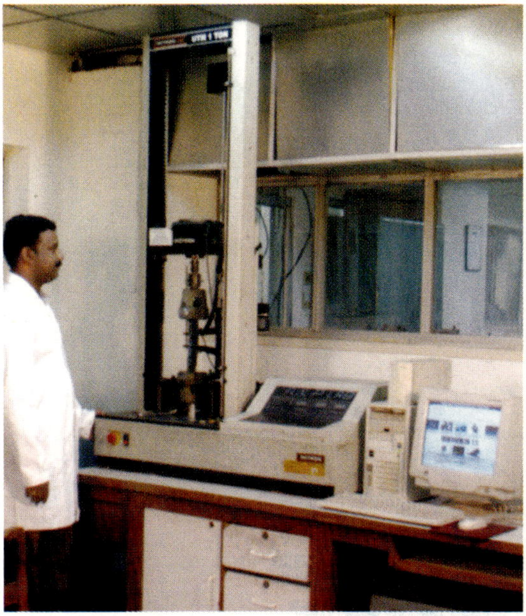

Mechanical testing of polymeric samples on Instron – UTM

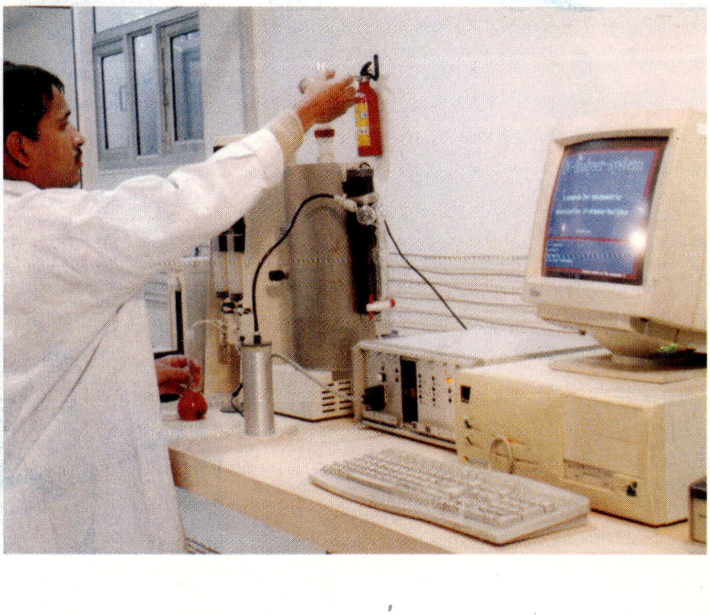

Adsorbable organic halides (AOX) analysis

Photographs Courtesy: Shriram Institute for Industrial Research, Delhi.

PLATE 2

KEEPING UNDER CONTROL THE TECHNICAL, HUMAN AND ENVIRONMENTAL FACTORS AFFECTING LABORATORY SERVICES QUALITY

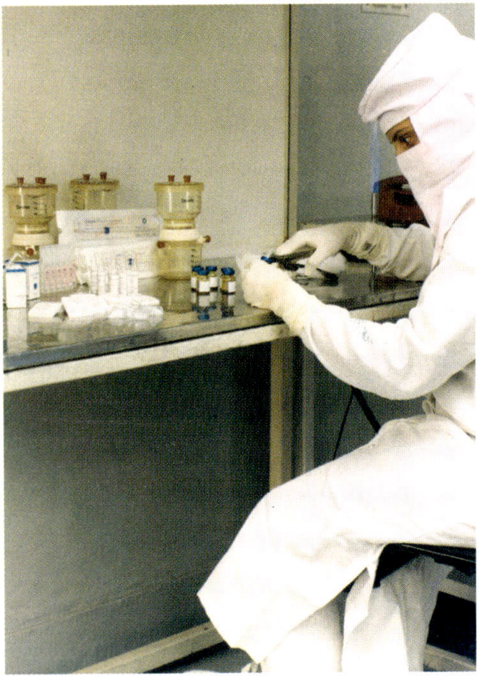

Sterility testing of injectibles using laminar flow in sterile room

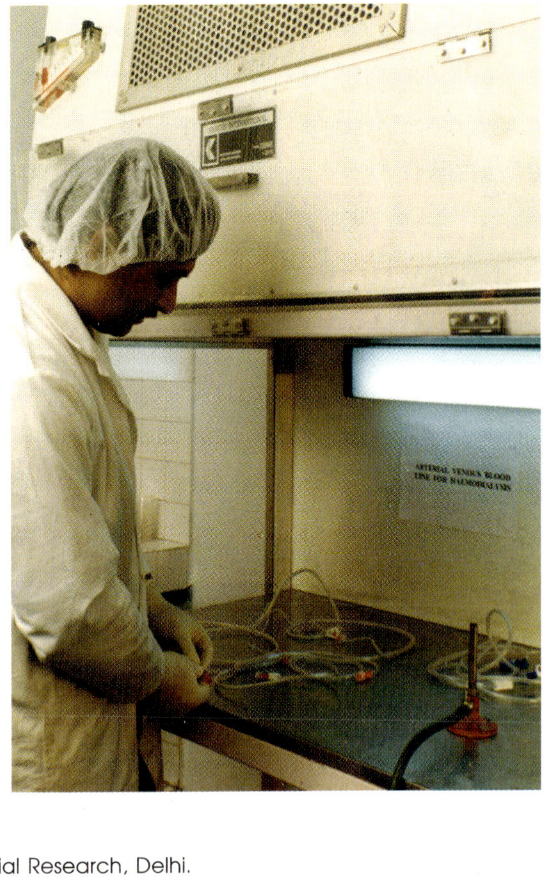

Sterility testing of arterial–venous blood line for haemodialysis using laminar flow in sterile room

Photographs Courtesy: Shriram Institute for Industrial Research, Delhi.

MOVING BEYOND QUALITY ASSURANCE: ASSURING BEST VALUE SOLUTIONS THROUGH QUALITY IN TESTING

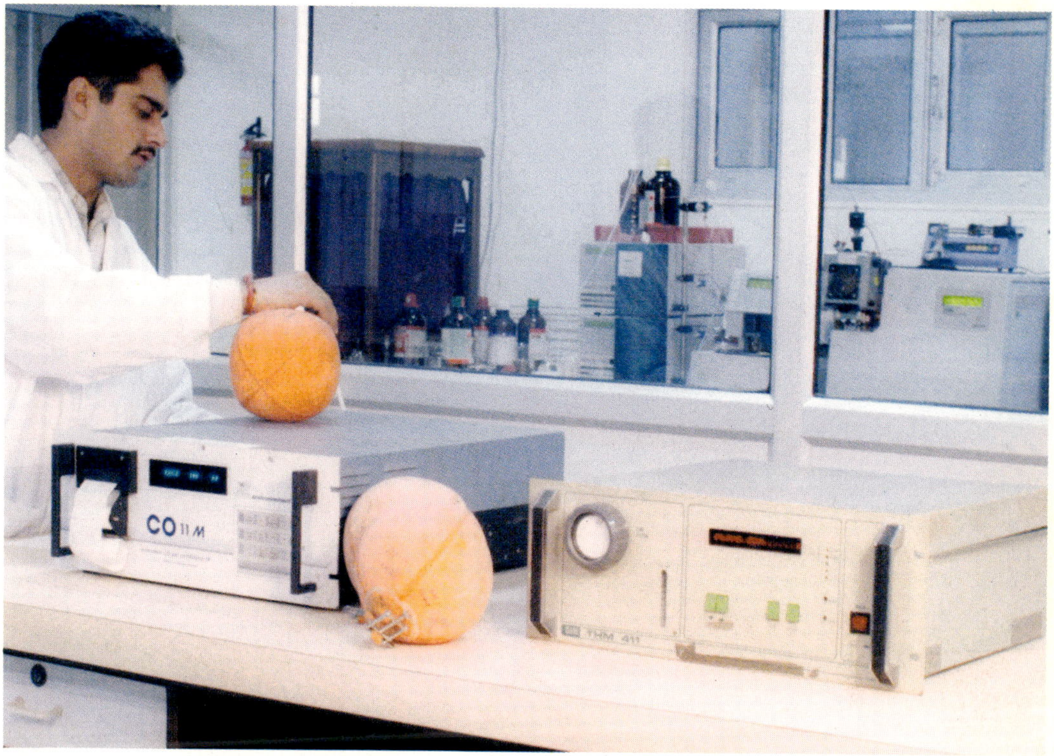

Carbon monoxide and hydrocarbon analysis of air samples from the industry

Photographs Courtesy: Shriram Institute for Industrial Research, Delhi.

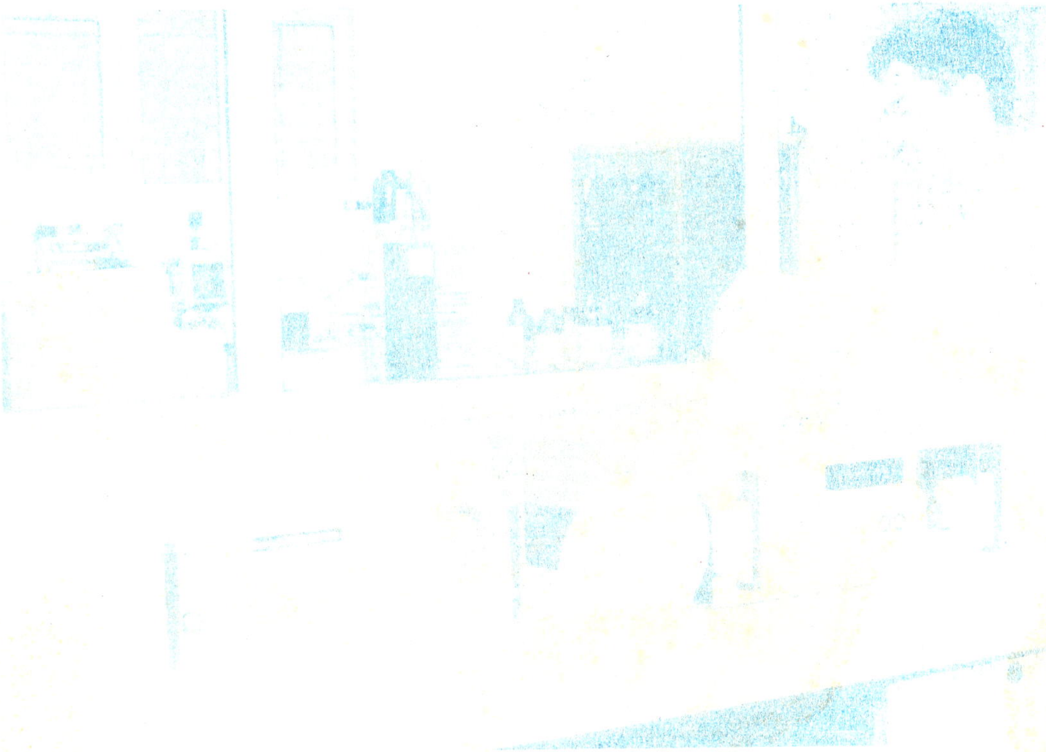

PART 1

Laboratory Accreditation

1

Introduction to Laboratory Accreditation

1.1 INTRODUCTION

It is well known that any business unit involved in manufacturing or production generally conforms its raw materials supplied by vendors to its own requirements through the standards established in-house. It may either accept the supplied materials as such or test its conformity in-house and be assured of the suitability for its own standards. Similarly the company may certify its product to its own standard. This is called a practice of self certification based on own specifications.

When a product certification body which is involved in product certification, certifies that a product conforms to the requirements of a specification, the consumer and the customer has a right to seek an assurance as to the competence of the product certification body. The credibility of certifying body is critically dependent upon the skill, expertise and professionalism of that body. Therefore, in order to provide confidence in the work of a certification body some form of recognition is required. Consequently it needs accreditation by a third impartial party. Therefore, the product certification bodies as well as Quality Management Systems certification bodies do need to go for the accreditation of their own competence.

It is possible to define accreditation as a process that generally applies to individuals, organizations and involves determination of elements of conformance to standards, judgement of competence, expertise and professionalism, and results in official recognition.

The accreditation of a certifying body is carried out by nationally recognized bodies such as Registrar Accreditation Board in America, National Accreditation Council for Certifying Bodies (U.K.), and Joint Accreditation System of Australia and New Zealand.

Thus when a certifying body is a *laboratory accreditation body*, its own accreditation must include an evaluation of scientific expertise and competence of its laboratory accreditation staff. When an accreditation body itself goes for accreditation of its own systems, the competence of its auditors or assessors is also judged. Therefore, an accreditation body must maintain its accreditation system through bilateral or multilateral mutual recognition agreements with other accreditation bodies of national or international standing. When a national level accreditation body has fulfilled the requirements of Mutual Recognition Agreement with another accreditation body at international level, the laboratories accredited under its aegis stand to gain acceptance of their test or calibration results by the concerned countries. This facilitates acceptance of the goods being traded with out subjecting them to retesting at the place of their end use.

1.2 MEANING OF LABORATORY ACCREDITATION

ISO Guide 2:1991 clearly provides a definition of laboratory accreditation. According to that it is "a formal recognition that a laboratory is competent to carry out a Specific Test or Specific Types of Tests."

Laboratory accreditation can not be a guarantee for each and every test result produced by an accredited laboratory. It is not a magical formula for closed eyed assurance. The laboratory accreditation is concerned with determining the ability of a laboratory to obtain a valid measurement data in a reliable way. In other words, the end result of accreditation is low level of uncertainty which reflects in high degree of confidence in the test or calibration results.

1.3 NEED FOR OBTAINING LABORATORY ACCREDITATION

The laboratories involved in testing or calibration provide reports of measured data to the clients for their acceptance either inland or abroad. The acceptance of the concerned report specifically rests with the accepting party. In case of disagreement over the results another laboratory may be approached to carry out the test or calibration on the same sample. In order to overcome such cases of dissatisfaction and to facilitate world trade, acceptance of test or calibration results is essential within or outside the country. Therefore, it is normal practice that laboratories involved in test or calibration are expected to demonstrate their compliance with national regulations or international guidelines.

1.4 AGENCIES WHICH PROVIDE LABORATORY ACCREDITATION

Laboratory accreditation is provided by a national or international accreditation body who has its own system of accreditation based on ISO Guide 58 : 1993 (Operation of Accreditation Bodies). The national laboratory accreditation body providing accreditation to test or calibration laboratories should itself have complied with requirements of a Mutual Recognition Agreement with other international laboratory accreditation bodies.

Any national accreditation body always operates accreditation system on *voluntary* and *nondiscriminatory* basis.

1.5 ESSENTIAL ELEMENTS OF LABORATORY ACCREDITATION

The laboratory accreditation generally covers the general requirements of accreditation as mentioned in ISO/IEC Guide 25: (1990). The national accreditation body formulates its own accreditation criteria based on these guide lines which is adopted as standard to be implemented by the test or calibration laboratories.

The accreditation body also publishes specific criteria dealing with a particular area of testing or calibration. Thus accreditation elements cover general requirements and specific requirements as stipulated in the accreditation criteria of a particular discipline of testing or calibration. However, the general accreditation requirements mentioned in the ISO/IEC Guide 25:1990 for laboratory accreditation cover the following :

- Organization Management
- Quality System Audit and Review
- Personnel
- Accommodation and Environment
- Equipment and Reference Material
- Measurement Traceability and Calibration
- Calibration and Test Method
- Handling of Test and Calibration item
- Records
- Subcontracting of calibration or testing
- Outside Support Service
- Complaints
- Relation with accreditation body

1.5.1 Specific Criteria Requirements

The Specific Criteria for different disciplines of testing or calibration are formulated by the national accreditation body covering the requirements mentioned under clauses and sub-clauses of general requirements of ISO/IEC Guide 25 (1990). The test or calibration laboratory seeking accreditation will have to address these requirements in its quality manual, wherever necessary. The sample requirements of Specific Criteria of Chemical Testing Laboratories are given below for understanding of the applicant laboratories.

- Scope
- Staff
- Environment
- Equipments
- Reagents
- Method/procedures for calibration and tests
- Calibration and measurement traceability
- Reference Material and Chemical Standards
- Use of Computers
- Laboratory audit and review

- Sampling, sample handling and preparation
- Quality Control
- Measurement Uncertainty
- Test Method Validation

1.6 REFERENCE TO LABORATORY ACCREDITATION GUIDES

International Organization for Standardization (ISO) and International Electro-technical Commission (IEC) together form a system for worldwide standardization as a whole, and publish various ISO/IEC Guides on laboratory accreditation on requests arising from International Laboratory Accreditation Cooperation (ILAC).

Some of the main guides are listed below for the information of laboratories seeking accreditation from national accreditation bodies.

Guide	Title
ISO/IEC Guide 2:1991	General Terms and their definitions Concerning Standardization and Related Activities
ISO/IEC Guide 58:1993	Calibration and Testing Laboratory Accreditation System
ISO/IEC Guide 25:1990 (Superseded by ISO 17025:1999 Standard)	General Requirements for Competence of Calibration or Test Laboratories
ISO/IEC Guide 43:1984	Development and Operation of Laboratory Proficiency Testing
ISO/IEC Guide 49:1986	Guide for Development of Quality Manual for Testing Laboratories

1.6.1 Use of ISO/IEC Guides of Laboratory Accreditation

The foremost use of these guides may be as follows,

ISO/IEC Guide 58:1993

This guide is followed by the laboratory accreditation bodies, who formulate their own Quality Manual, Systems, and Procedures for Laboratory Accreditation. This guide can also be used to develop a system for mutual recognition of Quality Control Laboratories of an industry having sister concerns at different locations in or out side the country.

ISO/IEC Guide 25:1990

This guide is followed by the laboratory accreditation bodies or certification bodies for formulation of General Criteria for Laboratory Accreditation. It can also be adopted by the test or calibration laboratories functioning independently or associated with industries for developing, establishing and upgrading their quality systems.

Now, these requirements have been replaced by standards prescribed vide ISO 17025 (1999).

ISO/IEC Guide 43:1984

This guide is followed by the laboratory accreditation bodies or certification bodies for formulation of General Criteria for Laboratory Proficiency Testing. This can be used by the industries to develop inter- laboratory comparison within their sister concern industrial laboratories.

ISO/IEC Guide 49:1986

This guide is adopted by the test or calibration laboratories or laboratories associated with industries to develop their quality manuals.

1.7 CANDIDATES FOR LABORATORY ACCREDITATION

Any test or calibration laboratory involved in repetitive nature of testing or calibration can avail accreditation from a national or international laboratory accreditation body. As per International Laboratory Accreditation Cooperation's recommendations the research laboratories, apex metrological institutions and laboratories to be recognized for Good Laboratory Practices are not covered under accreditation at present.

1.8 BROAD VIEW OF THE ACCREDITATION

The testing or calibration laboratories, while planning to get their laboratory accredited from a national or international accreditation body should inquire from the accreditation body about :

1. Testing or calibration areas covered by the accreditation body
2. Availability of Laboratory Accreditation Criteria
3. Specific Criteria prescribed by the accreditation body for the relevant area of testing or calibration
4. Assessment Criteria followed by the accreditation body
5. Expenses charged by the accreditation body for processing and accreditation procedure
6. Status of accreditation body in respect of Mutual Recognition Agreements
7. Nature of quality documentation required for processing the request for accreditation

1.8.1 On receiving relevant information as suggested above, the applicant laboratory should approach the accreditation body for obtaining the documents such as accreditation criteria, application form, Specific Criteria, Assessment Criteria, norms for expenses so as to start preparing for formally seeking the accreditation.

1.8.1.1 The applicant laboratory should submit the quality documentation such as laboratory's Quality Manual, application form along with accreditation charges to the accreditation body for examining the compliance of Quality Manual and technical requirements sought by application form.

1.8.2 The accreditation body, on scrutinizing the compliance of quality documentation to its accreditation criteria, normally organizes a pre-assessment. In this event the representatives of the accreditation body, generally called lead assessors/ lead auditor, ascertain the technical experts needed, number of man days expected, mode of payment of accreditation charges and readiness of the laboratory for on the spot assessment. The pre-assessment findings are submitted to the accreditation body for taking a decision on the assessment schedule.

1.8.3 For the purpose of carrying out initial assessment the accreditation body nominates technical experts of sound technical knowledge of testing or calibration areas for which the applicant laboratory has sought accreditation. The technical experts must have knowledge of rules, regulations, procedures, and accreditation systems prescribed by the accreditation body. The audit team consisting the lead auditor, technical experts etc. pays visit to the applicant laboratory for a prefixed duration of two to three days for on the spot initial assessment and interacting with the laboratory management and technical personnel to find out the compliance and effective implementation of the accreditation requirements as documented in Quality Manual of the laboratory.

1.8.3.1 The audit team, based on objective evidences, confirms the implementation of laboratory's generic accreditation criteria requirements as well as Specific Criteria requirements of a particular area of testing or calibration. The audit team prepares its assessment report and makes its recommendations for considering the applicant laboratory for accreditation. A copy of the report is handed over to the laboratory. The report is sent to the accreditation body for examination with respect to requirements of accreditation. The observations of the accreditation body are then sent to the laboratory for further follow up action in case the assessment report indicates noncompliance to accreditation criteria.

1.8.4 The assessment reports, on compliance with the accreditation requirements, are evaluated by the concerned evaluation panels consisting of technical experts having the knowledge of testing or calibration in the same area in which accreditation is sought by the applicant laboratory. The recommendations to accord accreditation, if given by the evaluation panels are considered recommendations only and the final accreditation is granted by the chairman/president of the national accreditation body. The national accreditation body issues certificate and the details of accreditation to the applicant laboratory and admits the laboratory to a directory of the laboratories accredited by the body. Thereby the laboratory is also authorized to use the logo of accreditation body on its test or calibration reports or advertising materials.

The flow scheme of stages of preparation for accreditation, grant and renewal is at Fig 1.1.

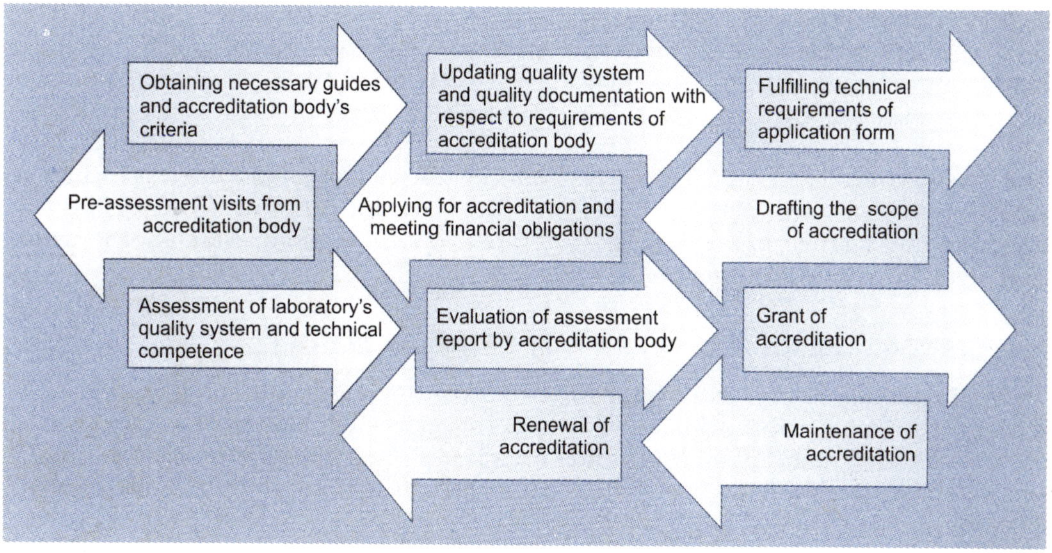

Fig 1.1: *Flow scheme of stages of preparation for accreditation, grant and renewal*

1.9 TECHNICAL REQUIREMENTS OF APPLICATION

The applicant testing or calibration laboratories while seeking accreditation from a laboratory accreditation body will have to provide the technical information about availability of equipments, instruments, testing or calibration personnel, nature of tests or calibration parameter to be included as accreditation details in the certificate of accreditation. This information may be detailed as mentioned in the sub-clauses.

1.9.1 The applicant laboratory should try its best to provide the equipment, instrument details for its make, model, purchase date, location range and accuracy of test or calibration equipment and latest calibration status.

1.9.2 The applicant test or calibration laboratory should ensure that the test or calibration personnel involved in testing or calibration meet the requisite qualifications, experience, and training in accordance with the requisite requirements of respective Specific Criteria for respective area of testing or calibration.

1.9.3 It is experienced that most of the applicant laboratories face problems while drafting the scope of accreditation. The laboratories are not clear on what is to be given and what is not to be given. Some times the laboratories mention the product specifications as their scope of accreditation which is not the correct way of drafting the scope. Sometimes they mention the test range and accuracy of equipment and name of equipment operation manuals as test method specification.

1.9.3.1 The laboratory accreditation is only concerned with the competence of laboratory to conduct a specific type of test or calibration. Therefore, the scope of accreditation should be related only to the test or calibration performed by the laboratory. The laboratory, while drafting its scope of accreditation should mention the nature of test being performed on a material or product, established test range and accuracy along with test method specification number. It should not mention test range or accuracy being given in a product specification.

1.9.4 The laboratory should carefully mention the validated test method when it uses its own developed methods based on some scientific literature. The laboratory, if making any change in any test or calibration method, should validate the same before putting that into practice.

1.10 FINANCIAL OBLIGATIONS ON THE PART OF THE LABORATORY

The applicant laboratory, while applying to a laboratory accreditation body will have to bear certain nominal charges such as application fee, assessment fee, surveillance fee, accreditation maintenance fee, and renewal fee. The applicant laboratory should contact the accreditation body for knowing the admissible amount and mode of payment.

1.11 MAINTENANCE OF ACCREDITATION

Maintenance of accreditation is of utmost importance, therefore, the laboratory accreditation body should update or revise its criteria of laboratory accreditation, Specific Criteria for specific areas of testing or calibration, whenever there is any change in respective ISO/IEC Guide/Standards.

1.11.1 The accreditation body, on granting the accreditation to the test or calibration laboratory, should ensure its compliance through yearly surveillance of accredited laboratory for maintenance of accreditation.

1.11.2 The accredited laboratory can ensure the maintenance of accreditation through internal audits, intra-laboratory or inter-laboratory comparison. The accredited laboratory should review its quality system documentation to check if it is still complying with generic accreditation requirements and specific requirements as laid down in respective Specific Criteria.

1.12 RENEWAL OF ACCREDITATION

The accreditation is granted to a test or calibration laboratory for a fixed period, generally three or five years duration, and its continuity maintained through surveillance as per policy of the accredited body.

The accreditation of a test or calibration laboratory is acquired on voluntary basis and for its continuation also depends on the will of the accredited laboratory. Before the expiry of the tenure of accreditation the accredited laboratory should approach the accreditation body with a request for its renewal. The accreditation body generally intimates the accredited laboratory prior to expiry of the accreditation period and requests for submission of latest quality documentation and accreditation fee so as to plan and conduct a full-fledged reassessment for the compliance with the accreditation requirements.

After confirming through evaluation of the audit reports of this reassessment for 100% compliance with the requirements of accreditation, the accreditation body intimates the accredited laboratory about the grant of renewal of accreditation for a fixed duration. The accreditation certificate and accreditation details issued to the accredited laboratory are also endorsed.

1.13 ADDITIONAL ACCREDITATION REQUIREMENTS IN RESPECT OF ISO/IEC STANDARD 17025:1999

The ISO 9000 series of quality system certification includes elements for laboratory quality systems in ISO 9001, 9002 and seeks the compliance of these quality system elements from the laboratories associated with the concerned industries. The ISO 9000 auditors while assessing a laboratory in a company are only concerned with the quality system elements. This is because there is no mention of technical competence elements in the quality assurance standards. The technical competence elements of laboratory are such as technical qualifications, expertise of personnel in the concerned test or calibration areas, availability of appropriate and current test or calibration method, environmental conditions of the laboratory, samples handling, reference standards and their traceability, uncertainty of measurements, validation of laboratory's own test methods etc.

Thus a laboratory covered under quality system certification standards such as ISO 9001, 9002 can face difficulties for its recognition of technical competence. Thus to make ISO/IEC Guide 25 more exhaustive, now the elements of accreditation are aligned with ISO 9001, 9002 and ISO/IEC Guide 25 is superceded by ISO Standard 17025:1999.

The laboratories covered for accreditation under ISO Standard 17025: 1999 shall also be covered for recognition under ISO 9001, and 9002.

The additional requirements of accreditation mentioned under various clauses of ISO 17025:1999 are as follows:

- Document control
- Review of request, tendering and contracts
- Service to the client
- Control of nonconforming test and/or calibration work
- Corrective action
- Preventive action
- Internal audit
- Traceability of measurement for calibration
- Method validation
- Sampling

Cross references between ISO/IEC guide 25:1990 and ISO/IEC Standard 17025: 1999 are available for ready use at Appendix 1 at the end of this volume.

PART 2

Laboratory Quality System Documentation

2

Introduction to Laboratory Quality System

2.1 INTRODUCTION

The test or calibration laboratory while carrying out certain test or calibration needs to document the procedures as to how the samples of testing or calibration are collected, how the samples are handed over by the clients to the laboratory, how does the laboratory store or preserve the samples, how are the samples handed over to the analyst or test or calibration personnel, what tests or calibrations are to be followed for a sample, how are the test or calibration results to be recorded, and how is it to be ensured that the equipment/instrument will provide the correct and reliable results.

In the same way laboratory has to document the availability of reference standards and their appropriate condition, the procedures of equipment/instrument calibration, maintenance status and procedures to inform the clients about test or calibration results and complaint redressel. The ultimate aim of the laboratory is to satisfy its clients through appropriate documentary evidences being maintained for the policy and procedures followed in the laboratory.

2.2 MEANING OF QUALITY IN TEST OR CALIBRATION

The quality in test or calibration, is a conformance of the requisite requirements to a specification, or a standard fixed by the company for its product or materials to be manufactured. The quality in test or calibration is obtained by the concerned laboratory through use of well documented and specialized form of quality assurance system in the laboratory.

The quality in test or calibration is an important aspect for the satisfaction of its own internal and external clients. The quality in test is essential to provide safety to the human life, protection of health, buildings and to meet the national or international regulations. It can be said that appropriate and reliable test or calibration are results of quality maintained during various activities followed for sample's analysis or calibration.

2.3 SOURCE OF QUALITY IN TEST OR CALIBRATION

What key elements impart quality to test or calibration? If a laboratory has commissioned high precision and accurate equipments or instruments but has reluctance to employ the highly qualified, experienced and trained personnel, and bothers least to follow appropriate test or calibration reference conditions and adequate test or calibration methods, the results thus obtained may not be of the appropriate quality.

The foremost question before a test or calibration laboratory is - what is the mechanism to achieve quality in test or calibration performed? The quality in test or calibration can not be achieved only through the purchase of quality instruments, equipments and even employing the highly qualified test or calibration personnel.

The quality in test or calibration can be achieved if a laboratory gives thought to–

- selection of site for the laboratory
- design of laboratory building
- selection of instruments
- formulation of purchase specifications for instruments/equipments
- arrangement of integrated lighting system
- layout of laboratory instrumentation
- installation and commissioning of instrument facilities
- prevention of dust and vibration
- collection of specifications for test or calibration methods
- development of laboratory quality documentation
- mechanism for latest information on test or calibration method improvements
- external training to test or calibration personnel
- internal training (on-job) to test or calibration personnel
- following statistical quality control techniques
- development of control charts
- repeat and spiked test analysis
- intra/inter laboratory comparison
- instrument validation
- preventive maintenance and corrective maintenance
- periodical calibration of instrumentation

The quality in testing or calibration can also be introduced through improvement in soft quality i.e. quality of test or calibration personnel. The soft quality of test or calibration personnel means how do these personnel behave with each other, with laboratory clientele, with national or international test or calibration bodies etc. The soft qualities also include interest of the personnel in work, habits of learning new technical ideas, habit of working in a team, etc.

The other factors which affect the test or calibration quality are the emoluments received by the test or calibration personnel and the promotional avenues available to them. Addition of latest techniques for test or calibration can also improve the quality.

Therefore, it can be said that the laboratory quality management system organizes overall activities of the laboratory in such a way that technical, administrative and human factors affecting the test or calibration quality are under control. All such controls are oriented towards elimination, reduction and most importantly prevention of test or calibration quality deficiencies. The laboratory quality management system has to meet the interrelated needs of the laboratory and the customers.

The laboratory's needs are to attain and maintain quality test or calibration at optimum cost by efficient utilization of technical personnel, consumables and instrument or equipments. The customer's needs are to have confidence in capability of the laboratory to provide the reliable quality of test or calibration at competitive cost and maintaining the same consistently.

The laboratory quality management system puts into practice the cost effective concept of getting it right first time and every time. The laboratory quality management system starts with the identification of internal or external customer needs and quality requirements and ends only when the test or calibration results have been handed over to the clients for their acceptance or rejection.

2.4 ELEMENTS OF LABORATORY QUALITY SYSTEM

The Quality System in general, as described in the ISO/IEC Guide 8402:1987 (definitions) and ISO/IEC Guide 25:1990, states about the organizational structure, responsibilities, procedures, process and resources for implementing quality management. The generic requirements for laboratory quality system as stipulated under various clauses of ISO/IEC Guide 25:1990 (Fig. 2.1) are as follows –

- Organization and Management (clause 4)
- Quality System audit and review (clause 5)
- Records (clause 12)
- Subcontracting of calibration or test (clause 14)
- Out side support service (clause 15)
- Complaints (Clause 16)

These elements are briefly described here.

2.4.1 Organization and Management

The laboratory management shall clearly define the laboratory's legal status, its type, organization through organization charts, and management mechanism for protection of confidential information and rights of clients, and for independence of judgement.

2.4.2 Quality System audit and Review

The laboratory shall clearly define and document the quality policy, objective and commitment to quality of test and calibration services and good laboratory practices.

The laboratory shall formulate a quality manual, standard operating procedures, work instructions, forms and format for appropriate use of the laboratory.

The laboratory shall clearly lay down its policy and procedures for internal quality audits for each Quality System as well as technical competence element along with management reviews. The laboratory shall document its policy and procedures for various quality control checks for maintaining quality of test and calibration results.

2.4.3 Records

The laboratory shall define and document its policy and procedures for safety, retention period, storing conditions and security for original records for technical data.

2.4.4 Subcontracting of Calibration or Test

The laboratory shall clearly define and document its policy and procedures in case it subcontracts its test or calibration partially or fully to another laboratory. The laboratory shall ensure that the subcontracted laboratory does comply with the requirements of ISO/IEC Guide 25:1990.

2.4.5 Out Side Support Service

The laboratory shall define and document its policy and procedure for obtaining services from the outside suppliers for laboratory consumables, maintenance and calibration of instrumentation. The laboratory shall establish its own procedures for compliance of outside services, material and instrument/equipment to specified requirements.

2.4.6 Complaints

The laboratory shall define and document its system for internal and external complaints redressel.

2.5 QUALITY SYSTEM REQUIREMENTS

The Quality System requirements for laboratory accreditation as described in the latest ISO/IEC 17025:1999 standard of laboratory accreditation (Fig. 2.2) are as follows:

- Management requirements
- Organization
- Quality System
- Document Control
- Review of request, tendering and contracts
- Subcontracting of tests and calibration
- Purchasing services and supplies
- Complaints
- Service to the client

- Control of nonconforming testing and/or Calibration work
- Corrective action
- Preventive action
- Control of records
- Internal audits
- Management Review

2.5.1 Elements of Laboratory's Technical Competence

The test or calibration laboratories are currently required to follow the technical requirements as described under the clause of ISO/IEC Guide 25:1990 (Fig. 2.1) which are as follows :

- Personnel (cl. 6)
- Accommodation and environment (cl.7)
- Equipment and reference material (cl. 8)
- Measurement Traceability and calibration (cl. 9)
- Calibration and test methods (cl. 10)
- Handling of test and calibration item (cl. 11)
- Certificates and Reports (cl. 12)

The technical elements for competence of the laboratory are briefly defined as follows :

1. *Personnel*

The laboratory shall define and document that the technical personnel involved in testing or calibration are complying to the requirements of qualification, experience and specialized expertise in accordance with respective Specific Criteria of testing or calibration brought out by the national or international accreditation body.

2. *Accommodation and Environment*

The laboratory shall clearly define and document about the appropriateness of its accommodation, compliance with test or calibration environment conditions, and their monitoring and recording.

3. *Equipment and Reference Material*

The laboratory should maintain appropriate equipment, instrument, reference material, certified reference material, and secondary reference material for testing or calibration. The laboratory shall define and document its policy or procedures for maintenance of equipment and use of equipment which are outside its permanent control. The laboratory shall maintain records for equipments and their spares and reference material.

4. Measurement Traceability and Calibration

The laboratory shall maintain a programme of calibration, verification, and validation of equipment. The laboratory shall also maintain its measurement traceability to a national or international body. The laboratory shall ensure correlation of results through suitable inter-laboratory comparison or proficiency testing (in case traceability to national standards is not applicable). The reference standards shall be used for calibration. Only the reference standards shall be used for calibration. The reference standards shall be calibrated only by a laboratory who possesses an unbroken chain of traceability of measurement to a national or international body.

5. Calibration and Test Methods

The laboratory shall define, document and maintain standard methods of testing or calibration of items or samples. A standard operating procedures manual dealing with testing or calibration should be formulated. The laboratory shall use documented sampling procedures for sampling if it is a part of testing. It shall ensure use of validated nonstandard methods through agreements with clients for documentary evidences.

The laboratory shall ensure documented procedure for use of computers being used for capture, manipulation, recording, reporting, storage or retrieval of calibration or test data. It should also ensure security and protection of data.

6. Handling of Test and Calibration Item

The laboratory shall define, document and maintain a system for identification of items received for testing or calibration. It shall ensure appropriateness of received items for calibration or test. The laboratory shall document procedures to avoid deterioration, damage and safe storage, disposal, retention of test or calibration items.

7. Certification and Reports

The laboratory shall develop, document, implement and maintain format for test or calibration results covering technical requirement as stipulated in the ISO/IEC Guide 25:1990 or the latest standard ISO 17025:1999 for the laboratory accreditation. The laboratory shall document its policy and procedures for supplementing the incorrect test or calibration results already sent to the clients.

2.6 TECHNICAL REQUIREMENTS

2.6.1 The technical requirements as stipulated in the latest Standard ISO 17025: 1999 (Fig.2.2), which will have to be implemented by the laboratories involved in testing or calibration on demands from national accreditation bodies, are as follows:

- Technical requirements
- General requirements
- Personnel
- Accommodation and environmental conditions
- Test and calibration method and method validation

- Equipment
- Measurement traceability
- Sampling
- Handling of test or calibration items
- Assuring the quality of test and calibration results
- Reporting the results

QUALITY SYSTEM ELEMENTS	ELEMENTS OF TECHNICAL COMPETENCE
• Organization and management	• Personnel
• Quality system audit and review	• Accommodation and environment
• Records	• Equipment and reference material
• Subcontracting of calibration or tests	• Measurement traceability and calibration
• Purchasing services and supplies	• Calibration and test methods
• Complaints	• Handling of test and calibration items
• Outside support service	• Certificates and reports
• Complaints	

Fig 2.1: *Requirements of ISO/IEC guide 25: 1990*

QUALITY SYSTEM ELEMENTS	ELEMENTS OF TECHNICAL COMPETENCE
• Management requirements	• Technical requirements
• Organization	• General requirements
• Quality system	• Personnel
• Document control	• Accommodation and environmental studies
• Review of requesttendering and contracts	• Test and calibration method and method validation
• Subcontracting of tests and calibration	• Equipment
• Purchasing services and supplies	• Measurement traceability
• Complaints	• Sampling
• Services to the client	• Handling of test or calibration items
• Control of non-confirming testing	• Assuring the quality of test and calibration results
• And/or calibration work	• Reporting the results
• Corrective action	
• Control of records	
• Internal audits	
• management Review	

Fig 2.2: *Requirements of ISO standard 17025: 1999*

2.6.2 Cross references for laboratory Quality System and elements of technical competence.

The laboratory Quality System and technical elements as stipulated under various clauses of ISO/IEC Guide 25:1990 are mentioned hereunder for quick reference of laboratories.

Element	*Clause in ISO/Guide 25:1990*
Organization and Management	4
Laboratory's Legal Identity	4.1
Permanent Laboratory	4.1
Temporary Laboratory	4.1
Mobile Laboratory	4.1
Independence of Judgement	4.2
Confidentiality and Integrity	4.2
Supervision Adequacy	4.2
Improper Influence Confidentiality of clients, Proprietary Rights and Information	4.2
Technical Manager	4.2
Quality Manager	4.2
Nomination of Deputy Technical and Quality Manager	4.2
Inter-laboratory Comparison and Proficiency Testing Programs	4.2
Quality System, Audit and Review	5
Quality System Documentation	5.1
Quality Manual and Related Quality Documentation	5.2
Quality System Audit	5.3
Quality System Review	5.4
Reporting of Audit, review finding and corrective action	5.5
Quality Checks for results	5.6
Personnel	6
Qualification, experience and training of personnel	6.1
Evidence for personnel training	6.2
Training Records	6.3
Accommodation and Environment	7
Laboratory Accommodation	7.1
Laboratory environment	7.2
Laboratory environment monitoring	7.3
Effective separation for incompatible activity	7.4
Laboratory controlled areas	7.5
Good Laboratory House Keeping	7.6
Equipment and Reference Material	8
Use of equipment and reference material outside permanent control	8.1
Equipment maintenance and procedures	8.2

Element	*Clause in ISO/Guide 25:1990*
Equipment, Reference Material-	
Labeling/calibration status	8.3
Equipment Records	8.4
Measurement traceability and calibration	9
Test equipment calibration/and verification programme	9.1
Uncertainty of measurement and traceability	9.2
Inter-laboratory comparison/proficiency testing	9.3
Reference standards of measurement	9.4
Calibration Programme for reference standards	9.5
In-service checks for calibration and verification	9.6
Reference standards traceability	9.7
Calibration and test method	10
Documented instruction for equipment operation, test or calibration item preparation	10.1
Standard Test/Calibration Methods and procedures	10.2
Nonstandard methods	10.3
Validation of nonstandard method and client agreement	10.4
Statistical techniques for samples	10.5
Checks for data transfer	10.6
Use of computers	10.7
Documented purchase procedures and storage of consumables	10.8
Handling of calibration and test items	11
Documented system of identification of test or calibrated items	11.1
Conformance to standard conditions of test or calibrated item on receipt	11.2
Documented procedure for handling, storage environment of test or calibrated items	11.3
Disposal of test/calibrated items	11.4
Records	12
Record system and retention	12.1
Safety and security of records	12.2
Certificate and Reports	13
Calibration certificates, test report/test results	13.1

Element	*Clause in ISO/Guide 25:1990*
Certificate Details	13.2
Subcontracted test/calibration results	13.3
Standardization of Certificate format	13.4
Amendments to calibration/test results	13.5
Despatch of defective test or calibration results	13.6
Electronic transmission of test or calibration results	13.7
Subcontracting of calibration or testing	14
Subcontracted Laboratory's compliance with ISO/IEC Guide 25	14.1
Record of competence of subcontracted laboratories	14.2
Outside support services	15
Quality of outside support services	15.1
Documented procedure for conformance of purchased equipment/material/services	15.2
Suppliers Records	15.3
Complaints	16
Complaints redressel procedure	16.1
Audit against complaint	16.2

For cross references between clauses of ISO/IEC guide 25:1990 and ISO/IEC standard 17025:1999 the user may refer to Appendix at the end of the text.

3

Quality System Documentation

3.1 MEANING OF QUALITY SYSTEM DOCUMENTATION

Test or calibration laboratory involved in testing or calibration generally has to interact with the internal as well as external customer for the purpose of testing, inspecting or making some specific measurement on some item under certain test reference conditions of a specification as mentioned by the customer in his request. The laboratory conducts the test, inspection, measurement and hands over the results to the customer, describing compliance or noncompliance of requirement to that specification. This establishes a relation between the laboratory and its internal or external customers.

The aim of the test or calibration laboratory is to provide reliable test or calibration data through a well defined, documented, implemented and maintained Quality System documentation. The aim of the customer is to obtain the reliable test or calibration data. Thus the laboratory carries out numerous activities to produce the technical data. If these different activities are put together, it constitutes a system. Thus, documenting these systems to produce quality test or calibration data can be termed as "Laboratory Quality System Documentation".

3.2 NECESSITY OF LABORATORY QUALITY SYSTEM DOCUMENTATION

The structure of laboratory quality management system is based on the concept of working together of a laboratory with its customer to analyze the test or calibration items in accordance with the specified requirements as stipulated in a specification to fulfill their mutual requirements. The customer's requirements are to secure confidence in the ability of laboratory to provide consistently reliable test or calibration data. The laboratory's requirements are to attain and maintain the reliability of the test or calibration data at an optimal cost by efficient utilization of technical personnel and facilities for test or calibration available to the laboratory. Therefore, the documentation plays a role in developing confidence in the customer and to secure consistency in quality of test or calibration data.

Let us take an example that a multinational laboratory, which has various laboratories located in different countries, conducts tests on a particular sample in all these laboratories to determine a particular characteristic. In such cases it is not necessary that the values obtained by all these laboratories are uniform and consistent. Therefore, a customer, before giving a sample to any of these laboratories, would like to have confidence that the laboratory is competent to produce the consistent and quality test or calibration data. At the same time, the laboratories in question are concerned to provide reliable and quality test or calibration data to meet the requirements of the customer to his satisfaction. In order to fulfill the mutual needs of the laboratories and customers it is of foremost importance that all these laboratories across the globe should have documented procedures for sample preparation, test or calibration method, test or calibration reference conditions, quality of reagents, equipments' accuracy, test or calibration personnel qualification and experience to achieve the consistent and quality results. More over a team of auditors should periodically visit these laboratories to find out:

- whether the test or calibration personnel involved in testing or calibration are following a documented laboratory quality system (System Audit);
- whether this existing system is capable to provide quality test or calibration results (System Review).

If any deficiency is found out in the system/technical audit and reviews, all the laboratories should be advised to implement a uniform quality system so as to produce uniform and consistent quality in test or calibration results. This uniformity and consistency of quality in test/calibration results is thus produced through a documented system.

Therefore, in order to attain and maintain quality in test or calibration, a documented system is necessary :

- To provide interpretation and to avoid differing opinions;
- To provide permanent reference for maintenance and implementation of quality system;
- To create customer confidence in competence of the laboratory;
- To guide the laboratory for quality requirements of test or calibration;
- To train the laboratory test or calibration personnel;
- To provide a basis for audit and reviews;
- To facilitate changes in laboratory quality system;
- To act as a means of communication between the laboratory and its users;
- To meet the requirements of ISO/IEC Guide 25;
- To meet the requirements of latest standard ISO 17025:1999 for laboratory accreditation.

3.3 THE MATTER AND METHOD FOR DOCUMENTING

While formulating quality system for laboratories, most of the quality managers face problems regarding what and how to document. Many would think that purpose of documentation is to satisfy the ISO/IEC Guide 25 or the laboratory accreditation body. But in reality the primary objective of documentation is to achieve the quality in test or calibration which ultimately satisfies the customer.

There is no need to document every activity, and every procedure followed in the laboratory but the activity and procedure affecting the quality of test or calibration must be documented. The laboratories should document Standard Operating Procedures and validated non-standards procedures therein if the test method is used to test an item or sample affecting the human being. Therefore, the laboratories involved in testing of chemical, biological, clinical nature of samples must document the Standard Operating Procedures. The laboratories involved in testing of mechanical, electrical, NDT nature, if following the specification need not to document the test method as it will be a repetition. But laboratories of mechanical, electrical, NDT (industrial/medical radiology) nature, provided they follow a nonstandard test method for testing of an item, should have the method documented and duly validated.

The testing laboratories should document work instruction for operation of the sophisticated instruments, sample preparation, sample handling for test or calibration, if criticality is involved.

The calibration laboratories should document work instruction for calibration method and validation method, as generally calibration methods are adopted from reputed books or product specifications.

What and how to document can be decided by the personnel who are performing the test or calibration. Thus the best way to document standard operating procedures, and work instructions is to involve the test or calibration personnel having expertise and appropriate experience. Test or calibration personnel may be interviewed by asking why are they doing it and how do they do it. If there are better ways to do it then the procedure may be reviewed and modified.

While documenting standard operating procedures or work instructions, it is necessary to have a balance to include technical facts and practical aspects. But if the SOPs or work instructions are to be prepared by the experienced engineers or specialist it may elaborate more on how the procedure is performed.

But to achieve quality in test or calibration it is very much essential that the test or calibration personnel must know why it is performed and how it should be performed to achieve the reliable data. Therefore, documentation personnel must skillfully take both the aspects but to the required extent. The flow charts may also help in identifying the correct procedures.

3.4 DEVELOPING QUALITY SYSTEM DOCUMENTATION

Before commencing the writing of documentation, it is important to define the size category of the laboratory. The laboratories may be categorized as large scale, medium scale and small scale laboratory. A large scale laboratory may have its corporate office in a country and have laboratories in different parts of the country. The medium scale laboratory may have its all laboratories such as chemical, mechanical, NDT, electrical all under one roof.

A small scale laboratory may have a single laboratory such as chemical or mechanical testing laboratory. For facilitating documentation, such laboratory should divide the ISO/IEC Guide 25 : 1990 clauses in two categories –

- Clauses applicable laboratory wide
- Clauses applicable to specific responsibility

For example the laboratory wide clauses are :

• Organization and Management	Cl. (4)
• Quality System Audit and Review	Cl. (5)
• Personnel	Cl. (6)
• Records	Cl. (12)
• Complaints	Cl. (16)

The clause of ISO Guide 25 dealing with specific responsibility are :

• Accommodation and Environment	Cl. (7)
• Equipment and Reference Material	Cl. (8)
• Measurement Traceability and Calibration	Cl (9)
• Calibration and Test Methods	Cl. (10)
• Handling of Test and Calibration items	Cl. (11)
• Certificates and Reports	Cl. (13)
• Subcontracting of Calibration or Testing	Cl. (14)
• Out side Support Services	

Thus a practical and quick document writing process will require that all concerned test or calibration personnel should be involved in formulation of laboratory quality system documentation. Therefore, it will be more appropriate to distribute document writing task to the concerned section in-charge and supervisors of the laboratory. The quality manager must identify which section in-charge or supervisor should be responsible for what clause of the ISO/IEC Guide 25. It may be more appropriate that technical manager should document standard operating procedure and work instructions.

3.5 LEVELS OF QUALITY SYSTEM DOCUMENTATION

ISO/IEC Guide 25: 1990 or the latest standard ISO 17025:1999 do not define specific levels of quality system documentation for test or calibration laboratories. But in order to achieve quality in test or calibration, there are several individual activities performed by the personnel deployed in various section of the laboratory. All these activities are aimed to have the quality in test or calibration and to satisfy specific requirements of the customer. Such numerous individual tasks are interrelated to each other. Therefore, to accomplish the quality objective, it is necessary that there must not be any task left incomplete and at the same time there should not be any duplication of attempt. All these tasks must be performed in a proper sequence and with correct quality procedures.

In other words, the laboratory quality objectives, task sequence, task procedure and other related quality assurance activities must be identified, defined, documented and performed in well planned and time bound manner.

There are several ways to document quality system. As per ISO/IEC Guide 25: 1990 or ISO 17025: 1999 the latest standard on laboratory accreditation, the laboratory shall document the elements of quality system as well as technical competence. Accordingly it shall establish and maintain a quality system to fulfill the requirements of the guide or the standard in question.

Thus, the documentation means, the written procedures for all aspect of operation of the laboratory will be established and maintained. In order to meet the requirements of ISO/IEC Guide 25:1990 or ISO 17025:1999, for quality system and technical competence, all elements adopted by the laboratory for quality management should be documented in the form of written policy and procedures.

The quality system is normally documented through a quality manual.

The Quality Manual states the quality policy, quality system and quality practices of an organization. The laboratory Quality Manual may be supported by several tiers of documents, each tier will be in more detail. For instance in a four tier documentation it may have Quality Manual, Quality System Procedures, Standard Operating Procedures, and quality records. Together with these documents it completes the documentation of the Laboratory Quality System.

Development of quality system documentation is one of the most important activity of the laboratory. The quality system documentation may be developed in three tier or more levels depending upon the need. Generally the four levels of documents are as follows (Fig. 3.1):

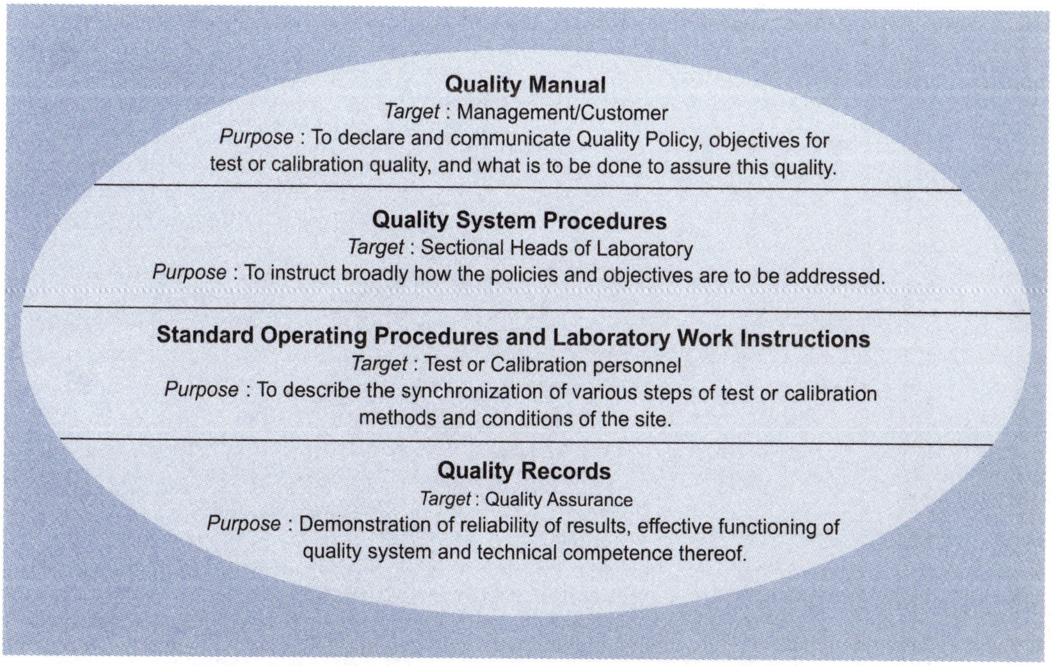

Fig. 3.1: *Levels of laboratory quality system documentation*

Level 1: Laboratory Quality Manual

Level 2: Laboratory Quality System Procedure

Level 3: Standard Operating Procedures (SOP) and laboratory work instructions

Level 4: Quality Records

The levels of laboratory quality system documentation are shown in Table 3.1:

3.5.1 The Purpose and Contents of the Quality Documentation

Quality Manual

a. Purpose To inform the test or calibration personnel and customers, regarding laboratory quality policy and objective for test or calibration quality. Specifically it states what is to be done to assure quality in test or calibration results.

b. Contents The Quality Manual must address each element of ISO/IEC Guide 25 or the latest standard ISO 17025:1999 for achieving laboratory accreditation. The elements need not be described in detail. The purpose is to assure the customer that laboratory has taken care to incorporate all aspects of the ISO Guide 25 or the latest standard ISO 17025:1999.

Users may refer to Fig. 3.2

Table 3.1

Level of documentation	*User/target person*	*Description of Documentation*	*Function of Documentation*
I	Management /customer	Quality Manual	To describe Quality System, Quality Policy, and laboratory accreditation elements per ISO/IEC Guide 25 or latest standard ISO 17025:1999
II	Sectional Heads of laboratory	Quality Procedures	To describe the individual quality activity in detail
III	Test/ Calibration personnel	Standard Operating Procedures and Laboratory Work Instructions	To describe the standard test/ calibration method and working instructions for laboratory activities
IV	Quality Assurance	Quality Records	To demonstrate performance of activity as per requirements of ISO/IEC Guide 25 or ISO 17025:1999.

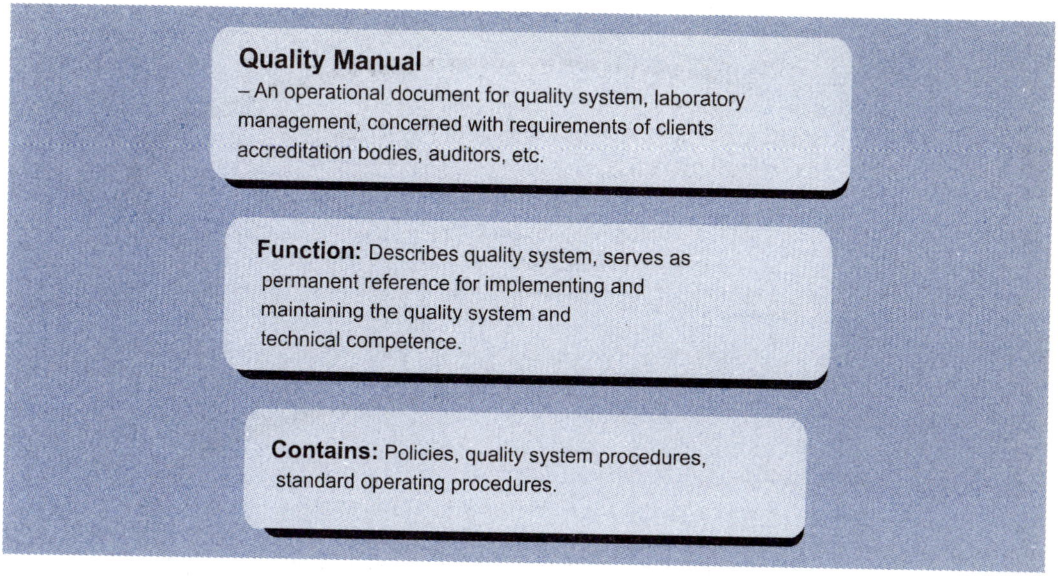

Fig. 3.2: *Contents, functions and purpose of quality manual*

Quality System Procedures

a. Purpose To instruct the test or calibration personnel in broad terms how the policies and objectives mentioned in the laboratory Quality Manual are to be addressed and achieved. Quality procedures are confidential document of the laboratory and can be developed separately for important activities of the laboratory.

b. Contents The quality procedures for laboratory, made to each of the statements of the Quality Manual, describe a systematic approach for all test or calibration personnel in same or different section so as to secure their collective efforts to meet the quality standard accepted by the management.

All the requirements of ISO/IEC Guide 25 or the latest standard ISO 17025:1999 should be covered. The quality system procedures should be made for all essential activities (Fig. 3.3).

Standard Operating Procedures (SOP)

a. Purpose Standard Operating Procedures are formulated to acquaint the test or calibration personnel about the synchronization of various steps of precise test or calibration methods with the conditions at the site. The SOPs formulated with involvement of the actual users is followed more easily by fellow employees.

b. Contents These documents are brief accounts of test or calibration method and describe the material needed, work involved in the step, data processing and evaluation, documents, samples to be stored and archiving instructions.

The scope, type and other features of Standard Operating Procedures are represented in Fig. 3.4.

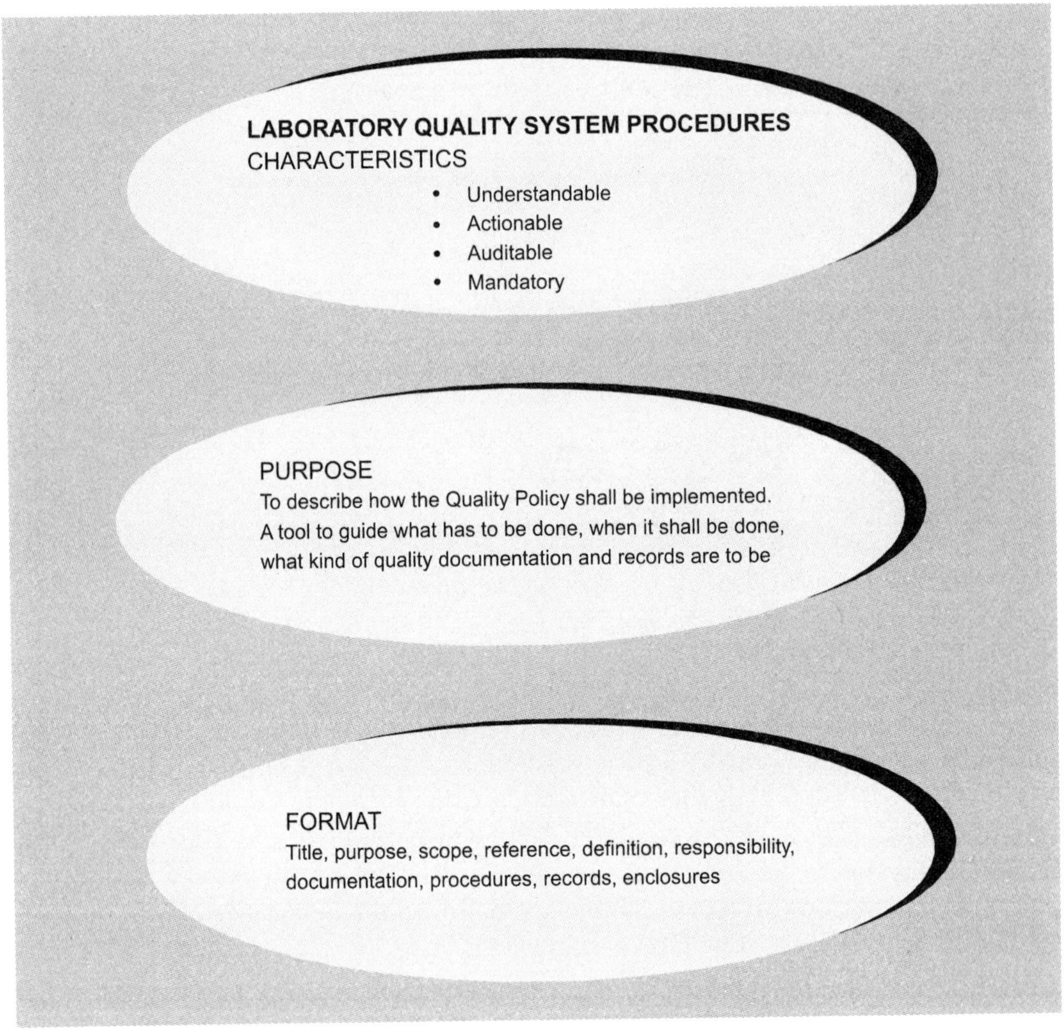

Fig. 3.3: *Purpose and features of laboratory quality system procedures*

Quality Records

a. Purpose To demonstrate that test or calibration results produced are reliable, and prove effective functioning of quality system and technical competence thereof.

b. Contents These include forms, format, test or calibration records, raw data, internal/external calibration records, maintenance records laboratory instrumentation and consumables procurement records, auditing records etc.

3.6 DOCUMENT CONTROL

In order to ensure that all test or calibration personnel involved in testing or calibration are using the same and correct version of documentation, it becomes necessary that quality system documentation is controlled (Fig. 3.5).

STANDARD OPERATING PROCEDURES

Cover - Administrative aspects, technical requirements, references of current specifications, standards, textbooks, etc.

Types - SOPs for testing, calibration, in equipments/instruments maintenance, cleaning, inspection, etc.

FORMAT

Numbering, title, name of test/calibration equipment, nature of materials needed, description of documentation, data processing and evaluation, documents and samples to be stored, approval and authorization, reference.

Fig. 3.4: *Scope, types and other features of standard operating procedures*

Document Control

Procedures for document approval and issue, change/modification, for

- Quality Manual
- QSP
- SOPs
- Audit and Management review records
- Test or calibration records
- Test or calibration data on computers

PURPOSE

- Providing document control irrespective of media
- Following established routine
- Ensuring appropriate updating of documents
- Ensuring use of authorised documents while implementing changes
- Avoiding confusion over multiplicity of sources, authorization of changes, issue of documents

Fig 3.5: *Document control and its purpose*

It is of much importance that which document is to be controlled as it will be difficult for the laboratory to control all the documentation used in the laboratory for various activities. This would require a record of who possesses the documents and a written procedure for the issuance of amendments and for reissuing, together with proper acknowledgment records. The documentation to be controlled can be described as follows :

- Quality Manual
- Quality System procedures
- Standard Operating Procedures
- Audit and Management Review Records
- Test and calibration Reports
- Test or calibration data on computers

The procedures of document control need to be established to address the following-

Document Approval and Issue

The laboratory should provide clear control of procedures and responsibilities for approval, issue, distribution and administration of documentation. The laboratory should ensure through its procedures that obsolete documents be removed in time and latest documents are put in use.

Document Change/Modification

The laboratory documentation may be subject to change, modification or revision, therefore, an adequate control should exist for the preparation, handling, issue and recording of changes. The laboratory should establish a mechanism for controlling changes in documentation. The controlling mechanism should have the under mentioned characteristics,

- Should provide control irrespective of the documentation media
- Should follow established routine
- Should ensure appropriate updating of documents.
- Should ensure use of authorized documents while implementing changes
- Should avoid confusion where multiplicity of sources, authorizing of changes and issue of documents are concerned.

Appropriate consideration should be provided to judge the effect of change on the procedure, which a proposed change will have on the test or calibration data quality. Action may be needed to assess the effect of change before implementing the same. The properly planned circulation of changed proposal among test or calibration personnel will avoid disruption. When a number of changes in documentation are to be coordinated the timing of implementation is an important factor.

3.7 DISTRIBUTION OF QUALITY SYSTEM DOCUMENTATION

The laboratory, before distribution of its quality system documentation either inside or outside the laboratory, should ensure that the required documentation is already categorized as controlled or uncontrolled wherever necessary. The test or calibration laboratory should always distribute duly marked controlled copies of Quality Manual to the accreditation body and respective authorized copyholder in the test or calibration laboratory. The laboratory should have a mechanism for controlling the distribution of documentation for amendments, revision, reaffirmation and retrieval of obsolete documentation from the concerned copyholder. For the distribution of documentation (Fig. 3.6), an appropriate numbering system should be followed by the laboratory.

3.8 MAINTENANCE OF QUALITY SYSTEM DOCUMENTATION

When quality system documentation is implemented for the first time in a laboratory, there may be instances that some of the test or calibration personnel will observe differences in certain procedures, test or calibration methods which may be an obstacle in achieving the reliable test or calibration data. The reasons for producing unreliable data can be detected by performing a series of tests or calibrations. On the

Distribution of quality system documents

Mechanism for *controlled* (for accreditation body and respective copy holders in laboratories) and *uncontrolled* (for clients, etc.) categories of documents

PURPOSE

- Control of distribution for amendments
- Revision
- Re-affirmation
- Retrieval of obsolete documentation

Fig. 3.6: *Purpose of distribution of quality system documents*

confirmation of the mistake or slip in the procedures, the matter can be brought to the quality manager or the technical manager for considering appropriate change in the quality system documentation.

It is possible that the laboratory might have applied for grant of accreditation to a national accreditation body and that body might have agreed that the Quality Manual conforms to accreditation requirements and conveyed so accordingly. However, it might so happen that on the visit for initial assessment it is observed that quality system documentation as prepared by the laboratory has numerous non-compliances and does not serve the basic purpose of accreditation. The laboratory in question will have to amend and reformulate its quality system documentation with a view to meet the accreditation requirements. The laboratory who has already acquired accreditation should maintain its quality system documentation and confirm its compliance by conducting periodic internal audits. On surveillance by the accreditation body, if certain deficiencies are observed in quality system documentation the laboratory should make changes in the quality system documentation. Also the laboratory should make changes in its quality system documentation if there are changes in accreditation criteria of the accreditation body.

Thus a laboratory should maintain its documentation through appropriate amendments, modification and revision to documentation for compliance of the same with latest changes in accreditation criteria also.

4

Laboratory Quality Policy

4.1 INTRODUCTION

The foremost aspect of implementing laboratory quality management system is a clear formulation of the quality policy and quality objectives. Any laboratory involved in testing or calibration cannot achieve the quality in test or calibration data without defining and establishing the quality policy of the laboratory. Thus a quality policy must be established to provide the limits within which all activities related to test or calibration are to be performed to attain the quality objective. The laboratory quality policy is a broad strategic pattern to guide and govern all laboratory management decisions towards the quality of test or calibration.

The quality policy of the laboratory is stated by the top management, as a formal and written document, in a manner that it is clearly understood by all the employees related to testing or calibration for the purpose of achieving the quality objective. Consequently the management gets an opportunity to express the quality objectives of the laboratory in the Quality Policy Statement.

This element plays a key role for the quality in test or calibration undertaken by the laboratory which ultimately satisfies the customer with the availability of reliable results. This means a business success to the laboratory and source of confidence for the employees. This stresses upon the fact that considerations of quality in test and calibration are of utmost importance as to the other policies also of the laboratory. This also stresses that each and every employee knows and understands his or her responsibility towards the laboratory commitment to test and calibration quality. Such type of quality policy provides guidance, as originating from the top of the organization, which ultimately shapes the quality procedures, standard operating procedures and other instructions with more details on the delegation of responsibilities down throughout all the operations.

The interrelationship of laboratory quality policy with quality systems and quality management in achieving test or calibration quality is shown in (Fig. 4.1).

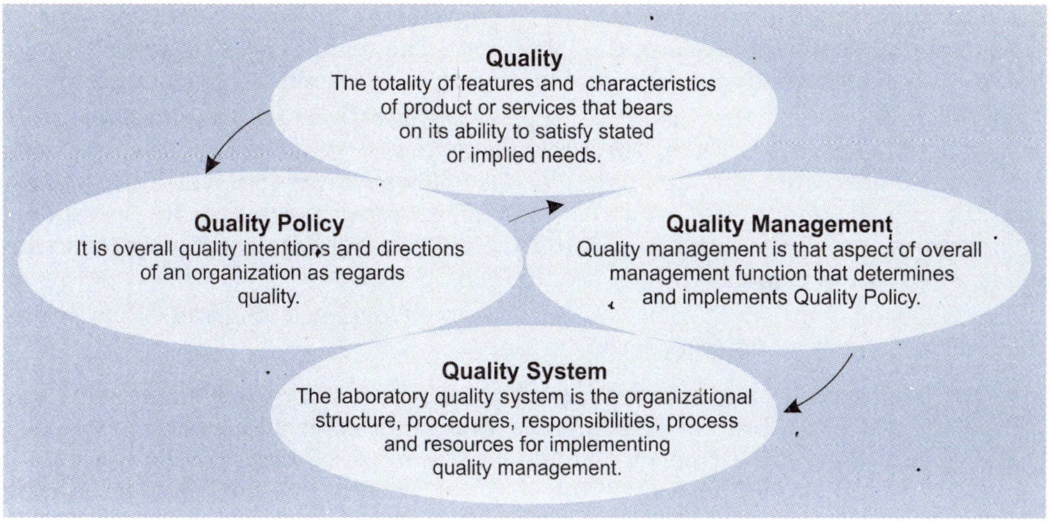

Fig. 4.1: *Interrelationship of quality policy, quality management, quality system and the quality*

4.2 LABORATORY QUALITY POLICY STATEMENT

The laboratory quality policy statement is of significant value as it leads all the ways to the management of laboratory quality. These ways are established specifically by means of each and every function of the laboratory in terms of appropriate decisions to customers and business. It will ensure that quality in test or calibration becomes the job of every one.

The laboratory Quality Policy Statement as signed by the top management is an important content of laboratory quality manual. The Quality Policy Statement should be known and understood by all test or calibration personnel involved in laboratory quality management. A properly thought out and prepared quality policy statement not only helps the laboratory in its implementation but also assists the laboratory in minimizing the errors.

4.3 DEVELOPING THE QUALITY POLICY STATEMENTS

The laboratory quality policy, as it is mentioned generally in quality manuals of various laboratories, appears as a policy fulfilling the requirements of product certification standards such as ISO 9001, 9002, etc. It appears then, that the laboratory concerned has not clearly deliberated or discussed this issue among the laboratory personnel concerned who are to be guided by this policy.

The test or calibration laboratories who are part of a large manufacturing organization should take care in developing their laboratory quality policy in that the laboratory policy will be different in some aspects from the company quality policy for quality system certification for its products. Therefore, it can be said that development of laboratory Quality Policy Statement and its objective is the job of a team. The laboratory should give appropriate thought while constituting the team to draft the Quality Policy Statement. The team should include the top as well as divisional and sectional heads of the laboratory. The team should draft the Quality Policy Statement and identify the quality objectives in support of the statement.

In the deliberations on this issue, representatives from all levels of laboratory management should be invited. The final Quality Policy Statement is a result of good and detailed deliberation in high places and is followed by an approval at the highest level. Though the intent is to involve all test, calibration and administrative personnel in development of the laboratory quality policy, the final statement and its implementation is responsibility of the top management.

The following points need to be specially observed for developing and documenting the quality policy and its objectives:

- The language used to express the quality policy should be easily understandable to the test or calibration personnel or internal or external clients.
- The laboratory quality policy should be relevant to the organization to which it belongs and should not violate the corporate quality policy of the organization in toto.
- The laboratory quality policy should be relevant to its other policies, services and laboratory personnel.
- The quality objective should be achievable.

The quality policy of various laboratories may vary because of their different nature of business or service but many things are common. Most of the quality policies, without any exceptions declare the intention of the laboratory to meet clients requirement against already laid down specifications and assure to provide the customer satisfaction. Few of the quality policies include a competitive language for test or calibration quality through a statement like "our test or calibration services comply to recognized specifications and provide more accuracy."

Many laboratories lay down their mission as continuous improvement in laboratory quality policy through a statement "Our laboratory will make continuous efforts to make improvement in test or calibration quality through adoption of latest instrumentation, analysis techniques and improved test or calibration methods."

Some of the laboratories associated with the manufacturing companies put an emphasis in their quality policies on "satisfaction of the internal customer".

Although there may be similarity in most of the laboratory quality policy statements but one should avoid to cut and paste quality policy draft from already published ones. Sufficient time should be devoted to define a realistic, practical and achievable quality policy which is most suitable to ones own laboratory. Thus the process of developing a laboratory's quality policy statement will provide an opportunity to demonstrate a new way of doing the things by involving test or calibration personnel more than usual and it will be beneficial to enlist the entire support from the very beginning.

4.4 OBJECTIVES OF THE LABORATORY QUALITY POLICY

During the last five years it has been experienced that most of the laboratories are mistaken about a clear cut demarcation existing between Quality Policy Statement and its objectives. Few of them resort to cutting and pasting the objectives of their company which has already obtained ISO 9001 or 9002 certification. This might serve as stop gap arrangement but in reality serves no purpose. A few others make no effort to describe the Quality Policy Statement along with quality objectives in their quality manual, and a few others make an ambiguous statute of the quality objectives.

It can be said that next step in test or calibration quality implementation process is the development of the quality objectives. The quality policy and the objectives need to be given importance in the right spirit of making quality efforts and essential, appropriate strategies must be developed to achieve the objective. The quality policy along with objectives must convey the intention of the laboratory on what it wants to achieve in reality (Fig. 4.2).

Every laboratory may have specific quality objective to suit its internal or external services. Few of the laboratory quality objectives which are generally applicable include and relate to the following (Fig. 4.2).

Compliance to Standards

The objectives relate to those features which provide confidence to customers on conformance of the laboratory quality system and technical competence to a recognized standard for laboratory accreditation.

Compliance to Specifications

This objective relates to what the test or calibration laboratory shall follow as duly approved, validated and recognized test or calibration methods for measurement or analysis as stipulated in specifications and have traceability to national or international body for measurements.

Test or Calibration Quality Improvement

This objective would include intention of the laboratory for improvement in test or calibration quality by using latest instruments and adopting improved test or calibration method if available.

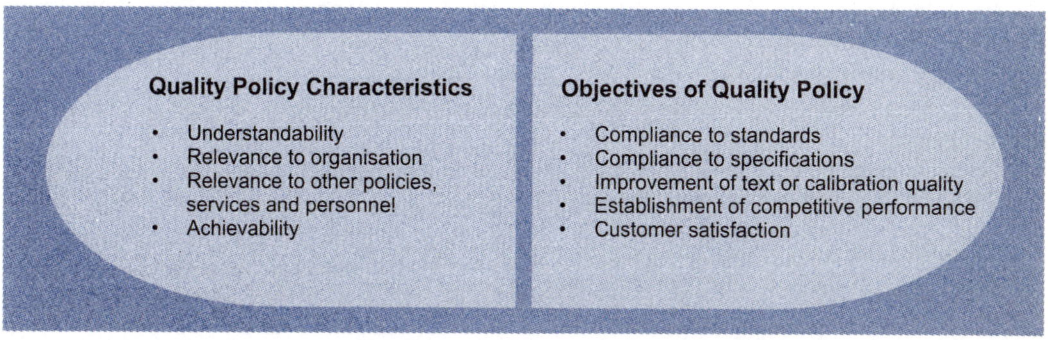

Fig. 4.2: *Characteristics and objectives of laboratory quality policy*

Laboratory Performance

This objective relates to those characteristics of the laboratory by which it establishes it competitive performance, through inter/intra laboratory comparisons, among its customers to avail more business.

Customer Satisfaction

This objective of the laboratory quality policy relates to those features of the laboratory which ultimately satisfy the customer with the quality of test or calibration results.

4.5 COMMITMENT TO LABORATORY QUALITY POLICY

Commitment to quality of test or calibration results is the responsibility of the top management of the laboratory. No laboratory quality system can survive without the commitment of the top management. The commitment that "we are going to implement whatever it is" is of no assurance of quality of test or calibration in any laboratory.

The commitment made by the top management for quality in test or calibration should be visible and stable on a continuous basis. The same can be demonstrated by,

- Requiring the laboratory personnel to understand and implement the laboratory quality policy.
- Initiating, managing and following up the implementation of quality policy and quality system in the laboratory.
- Not accepting any deviation from the laboratory quality policy.

The quality in test or calibration would not just happen but that has to be achieved through efforts of all, if they have good faith and discipline. If one has faith in the quality system, automatically he or she will be ready to acknowledge the positive results from the same.

Discipline is another element of the commitment. The discipline keeps the system in order, helps in formulation of appropriate procedures, and ensures involvement of every test or calibration personnel.

Commitment also means striving to be the best and to make efforts for continuous improvement. In other words commitment to quality improvement means a willingness to know the latest technical know how confining to the related areas around the world and to share the information in mutual interest.

The Quality Policy Statement of the laboratory must bear the signatures of the management.

4.6 EXAMPLES OF LABORATORY QUALITY POLICY

To elucidate the way of verbalizing the quality policy of the laboratory a few of the examples are mentioned hereunder (Example 4.1 and 4.2).

EXAMPLE 4.1

RAJSHREE TEST LABORATORY LTD.

Quality Policy

To provide testing and analytical services of recognized standards conforming to specific requirements for pesticides, effluents and water.

Policy Objectives

- To provide its customers at all times with a service complying with recognized standards of laboratory accreditation.
- To follow test and analysis procedures of recognized specifications.
- To maintain documents and records in accordance with laboratory accreditation criteria followed by the national accreditation body.
- To maintain the instruments and accessories to comply with the national standards.
- To manage the laboratory work with the staff having the necessary qualifications and experience with testing analyses procedures.
- To achieve finally full customer satisfaction with test results of the laboratory.

I declare to implement all necessary measures possible so that these policies are understood by each and every test or calibration personnel and ensure that every test or calibration personnel be involved and concerned by their applications. I assure that these objectives shall be achieved and sustained.

I have nominated Mr/Mrs ——— as quality manager to coordinate all activities related to implementation of these policies and for ensuring effective compliance of the same as stipulated in the current quality manual.

Signature

Managing Director, RTLL
RAJSHREE TEST LABORATORY LTD.

Place
Dated

EXAMPLE 4.2

BUREAU OF LABORATORY SERVICE

Quality Policy

BLS laboratories imparts services to its customers ensuring reliability, consistency and traceability of measurement of test or calibration data to national or international standards. BLS shall achieve and maintain it through –

- Regular maintenance and improvement in standard test methods by their periodic reviews.
- Instrument or equipment calibration on regular prescribed intervals.
- Need based test or calibration personnel training.

  Adopting new test methods.

I ensure that BLS will take all measures to implement all the policies as described in the current Quality Manual. Whenever I find any deviation from the stated policies, I will allow my Deputy General Manager (Quality Assurance), designated as Quality Manager and assigned the responsibility of quality system development, implementation and maintenance, to find the causes responsible for the same.

Signature

Chief Executive Officer
BUREAU OF LABORATORY SERVICES

Place:
Date:

5

Laboratory Quality Manual

5.1 INTRODUCTION

Laboratory Quality Manual is a prime operational document containing policies, quality procedures, and standard operating procedures of the laboratory, and it describes the quality system established by the laboratory management which serves as a permanent reference for implementing and maintaining quality system and technical competence.

For effective operation of the quality system it is important that the contents of the quality system as structured in the quality manual should comply to each and every requirement of the accreditation criteria being followed by a national accreditation body based on international standards.

The laboratory quality manual is a first level document which describes quality system in accordance with the stated quality policy and its objective for each of quality system and technical competence element of the accreditation criteria based on ISO/IEC Guide 25 or revised standard ISO 17025:1999 which is followed by the national accreditation body to accredit the test or calibration laboratories.

The quality manual contains reference of laboratory quality system procedures, a second level documentation used by the laboratory for quality planning and control of quality related activities. These quality system procedures become the basis of the quality manual and cover most of the elements of laboratory accreditation criteria. The quality system procedures describe the authority, responsibility, interrelation of test or calibration personnel and successive steps to perform a specific quality related activity.

The quality manual also contains the reference of standard operating procedures or work instructions, a third level documentation used by the laboratory to obtain reliable test or calibration data on following the appropriate, validated test or calibration method. The standard operating procedures are only concerned with test or calibration methods and describe the successive procedural steps to be followed for testing, or calibration of an item and calculation formulae or methodology to calculate the test or calibration results.

Quality Manual is a document concerned with laboratory management, clients, accreditation bodies and second and third party auditors where as quality system procedures, standard operating procedures and quality documents are mostly used by the laboratory personnel for its internal quality management.

5.2 DEVELOPMENT OF QUALITY MANUAL

A test or calibration laboratory, while developing a quality manual for its constituent laboratories involved in different areas of test or calibration, functioning from the same premises should develop a single quality manual for all those component laboratories.

If the laboratory is a part of some manufacturing organization already possessing a quality manual, then it should be restructured to align it with the requirements of the accreditation criteria. The modification should be made in the operative organization structure of the laboratory in relation to its parent organization.

The laboratory, having a number of its sister laboratories at different locations of the country should develop a laboratory quality manual for its corporate laboratory and separate quality manuals for all different laboratories. This can be done by appropriate modification in organization, scope of activities, job description etc.

To develop a quality manual, the first task of the laboratory management is to identify a suitable technical person with experience in laboratory quality system as well as laboratory management. The top laboratory management on satisfactory interviews, discussions, should nominate him or her as Quality Manager with a responsibility to develop quality system documentation and assure all the necessary documents. The Quality Manager should divide his or her responsibilities among the supporting personnel.

The responsibility of writing laboratory system quality procedures, standard operating procedures, work instructions may be assigned to different colleagues and can own up himself the responsibility to write the quality manual.

To commence the development of the quality manual he should document the existing operations, activities of the concerned laboratory and compare the same with the accreditation criteria. If comparison shows differences, then he or she would write policies and procedures as required for various quality system and technical competence elements as stipulated in the accreditation criteria of a national accreditation body. He or she should do best efforts that every element of accreditation criteria is addressed in the quality manual at an appropriate place.

5.3 WHO SHOULD WRITE THE QUALITY MANUAL

Document writing may be done by any one but quality document writing should be taken up only by persons who are familiar with the laboratory quality system and laboratory management. A technician or analyst who spent number of years in analysis may not be able overnight to develop a quality documentation. Thus the responsibility to write a Laboratory Quality Manual should be given to the Quality Manager along with assistance of supporting personnel or deputies.

6

Laboratory Quality System Procedures

6.1 INTRODUCTION

A procedure shows how the quality policy of the laboratory will be implemented, day to day, in specific areas and activities. A quality system procedure is therefore a practical tool to do an activity and to guide the test or calibration personnel. Thus the laboratory quality system procedures become the second most important part of the quality manual and that has a large bearing on the quality of the test or calibration. The documented laboratory quality system procedures are frequently used to plan and administer the quality related activities of the laboratory. Any quality system procedure associated with the laboratory should properly address all the elements in accordance with the accreditation criteria following ISO/IEC Guide 25 or ISO standard 17025:1999 for laboratory accreditation.

The quality procedures should describe:

- Appropriate control needed for the activity to be performed;
- Authority, responsibility, interrelationship of test or calibration personnel who manage, perform, verify, or review the concerned activity affecting quality of the test or calibration in question;
- How different activities are to be performed;
- Nature of the control and documentation required.

The documented quality system procedures denote the actual activities which have taken place in the laboratory at a specific point of time. Therefore, they should be subjected to evaluation and periodic reviews and changes to meet the demands or needs of the clients. Proper documentation, control and availability of the latest version of the updated procedures with the test or calibration personnel is very important for live and effective functioning of the quality system.

6.2 DEVELOPING THE QUALITY SYSTEM PROCEDURES

The development of quality system procedures does not only require familiarity with the concerned activity but also with different, successive steps involved in doing that activity. Thus in order to develop a quality system procedure for a laboratory, one should take care of the following :

- Quality system procedure must meet the requirement of accreditation criteria.
- Quality system procedure should contain all successive steps of the activity for which the procedure is made.
- Adequate involvement of staff to make the procedure practicable and successful.
- Adoption of existing documentation for records.

6.2.1 Development of Flow Chart of the Activities Associated with Quality System Elements

It is greatly helpful to precede the actual designing and documenting of individual quality system procedures with generation of flow charts for related functions or activities or series of activities required in the laboratory quality system. Users may refer to examples of such flow charts at Fig. 6.1 (Chemical test sample processing); Fig. 6.2 (Chemical sample calibration); Fig. 6.3 (Testing and analysis of medical sample) and Fig. 6.4 (Data calculation and analysis for medical diagnoses).

6.2.2 For writing such procedures a format should be developed by the test or calibration laboratory so as to ensure uniformity in all quality procedures. This format should include the following aspects:

Laboratory's Name:	QUALITY SYSTEM PROCEDURE	LQSP NO.
	TITLE: Laboratory Quality System Procedure Preparation	Revision:
		Page:

1. ***Numbering*** A numbering system allows for accurate cross referencing and integration of the separate procedures into a whole system i.e. Laboratory Quality System Procedures Manual. Many kinds of numbering systems are possible and none is intrinsically superior to the rest.
2. ***Title*** The title of a quality system procedure should be necessarily given to distinguish it from others.
3. ***Purpose*** Every quality system procedure must have its purpose and to make that explicit is a good discipline. It also aids implementation. Staff then knows why the procedure is followed. The purpose statement should be brief and clear as it is a bridge to the policy statement and therefore to the requirements of accreditation.

4. ***Scope*** The scope of a quality system procedure indicates the place in laboratory where it is to be applied. This might be described in terms of a section (e.g. sample receipt section), or activity (e.g. procurement of consumables, raw data), or analysis, or testing, or in terms of quality system itself (e.g. internal audit or management review). Making the scope explicit helps the practical implementation and test or calibration personnel.
5. ***Reference*** While carrying out a procedure, necessity might be felt to consult other instructions or guidelines. These may be internal or external to the laboratory quality system. Therefore, in case of interface of the quality system procedure with any other specific procedure or quality system document, a reference must be provided for the same.
6. ***Definition*** The quality system procedures should be written in simple, clear and understandable language, however, some times it is essential to use a term which is not understood by every one who is involved in use of the procedure. Most commonly this might be a technical term and should be briefly described by means of a formal definition in the procedure.
7. ***Responsibility*** The responsibility for implementing the procedure to achieve the purpose is to be defined very clearly.
8. ***Documentation*** The quality system procedure must be auditable and therefore objective evidences are required that the procedure has been followed. Generally this require documentation. This can be of various sorts (including electronic data). But in most systems documentation means forms and formats to record the data.
9. ***Procedures*** The procedure should be written in a short paragraph in successive steps, perhaps with numbering and subtitling so that the reader can quickly understand. All the activities should be written in logical way, clearly defining the responsibilities of the persons associated.
10. ***Records*** It should be clearly identified that which records are generated by using the respective quality system procedure, who is going to maintain the records and what will be its retention period.
11. ***Appendix*** Document like graph of test data or any other appended document as part of the quality system procedure should be identified as such.

Prepared by	Approved by	Date of issue

6.3 THE ESSENTIAL FEATURES OF A QUALITY SYSTEM PROCEDURE

The quality procedure as referenced in the quality manual should be described in detail. Each element of laboratory quality system or technical competence has its own set of quality procedure. These procedures are not just work of literature, they must be effective. To be effective they should qualify four tests.

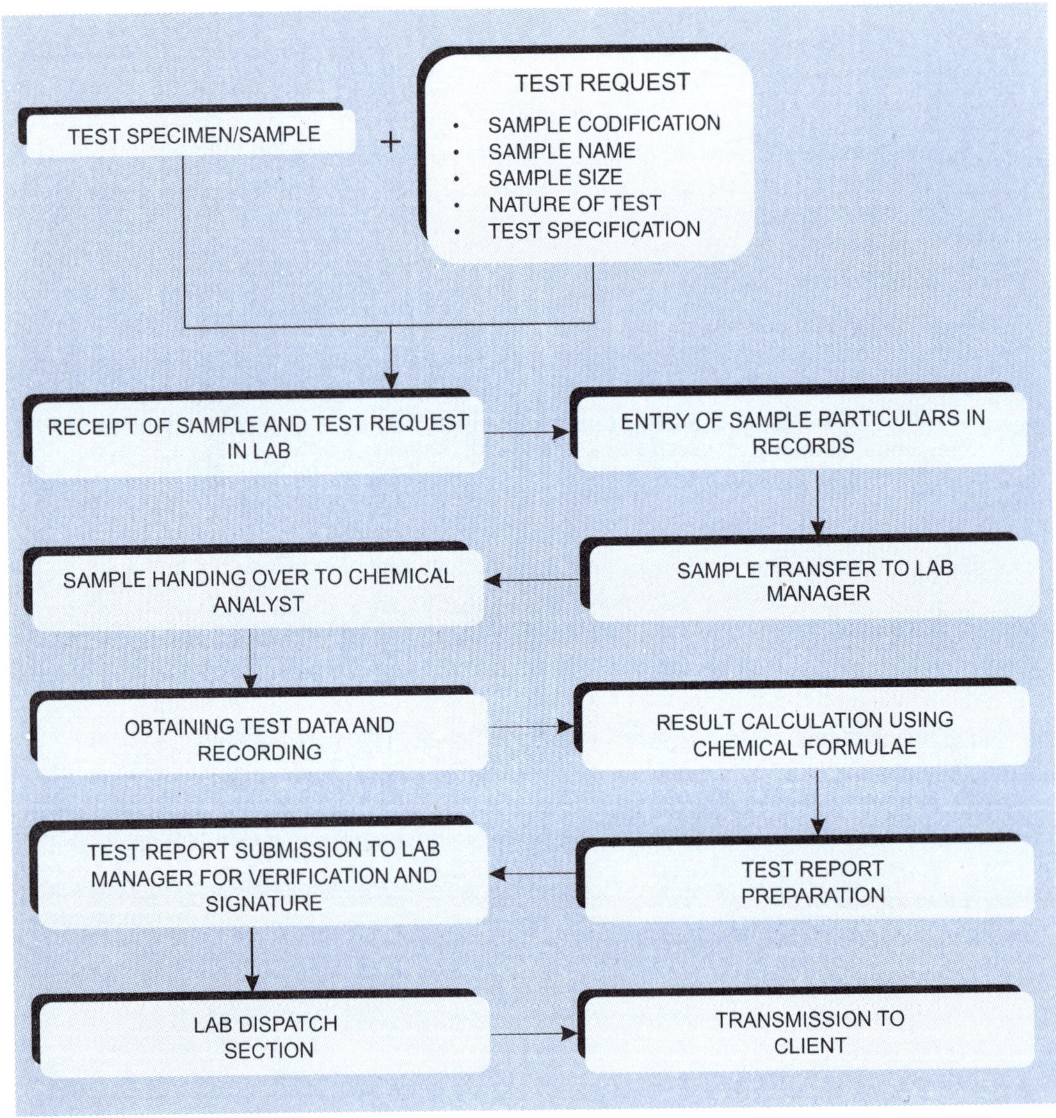

Fig. 6.1: *Flow chart for chemical test sample processing*

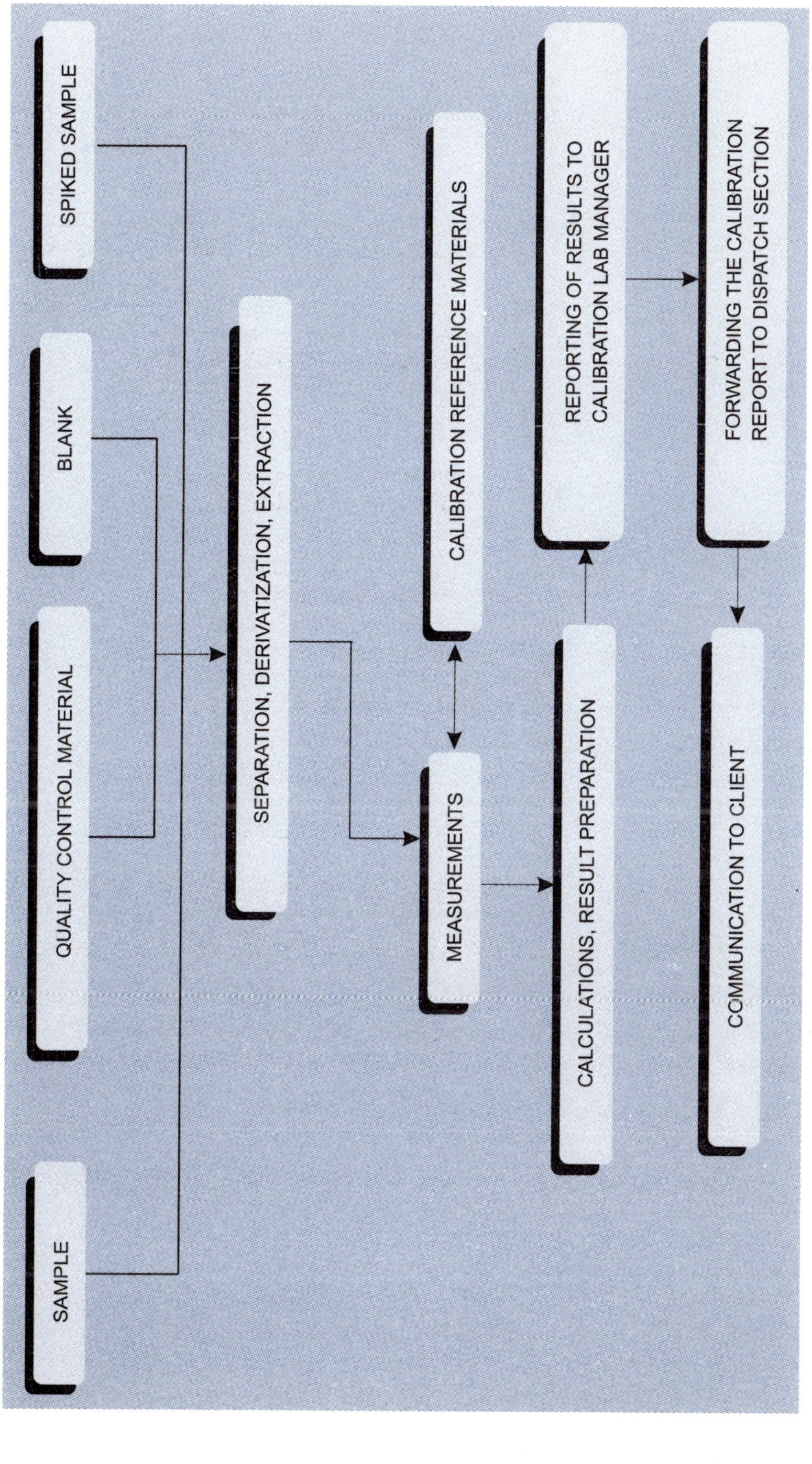

Fig. 6.2: *Flow chart for chemical sample calibration*

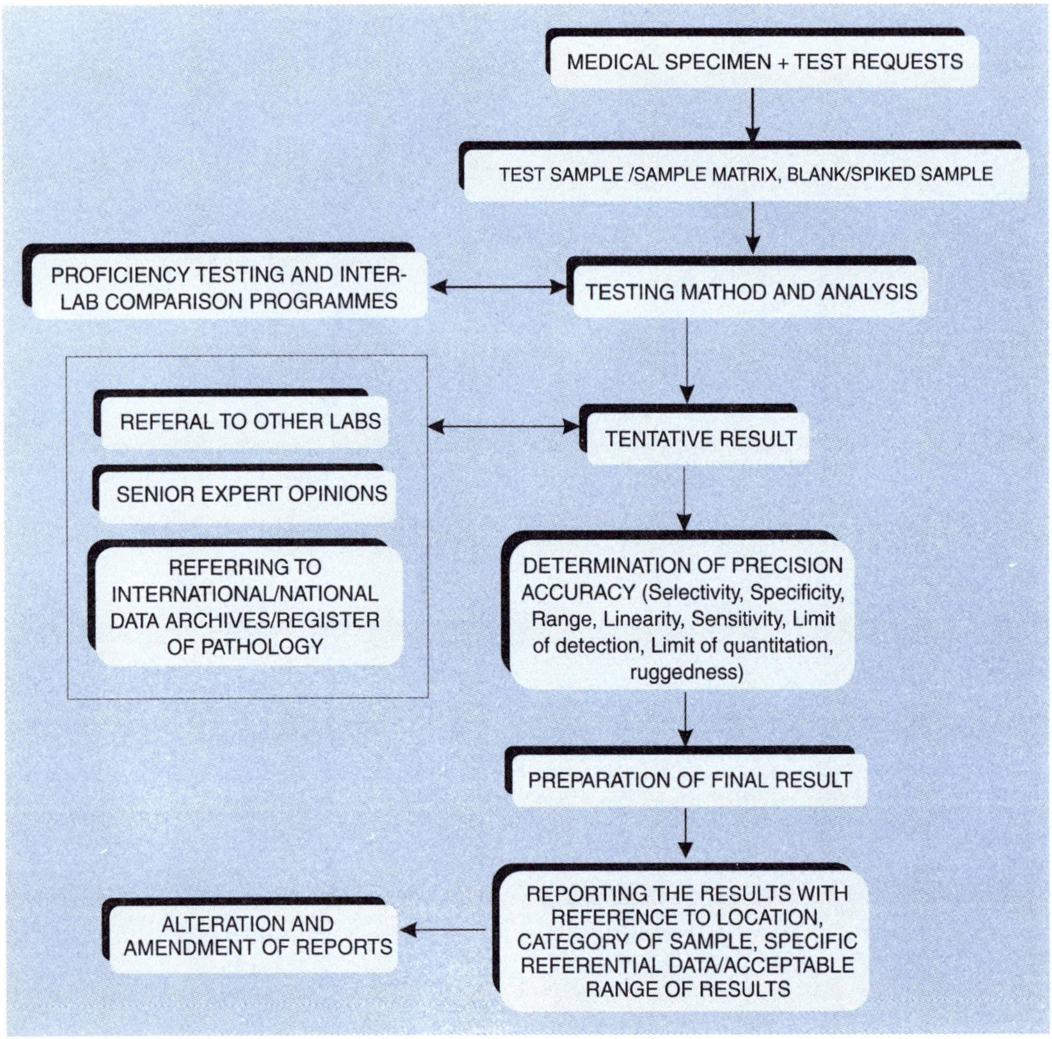

Fig. 6.3: *Testing and analysis of medical sample*

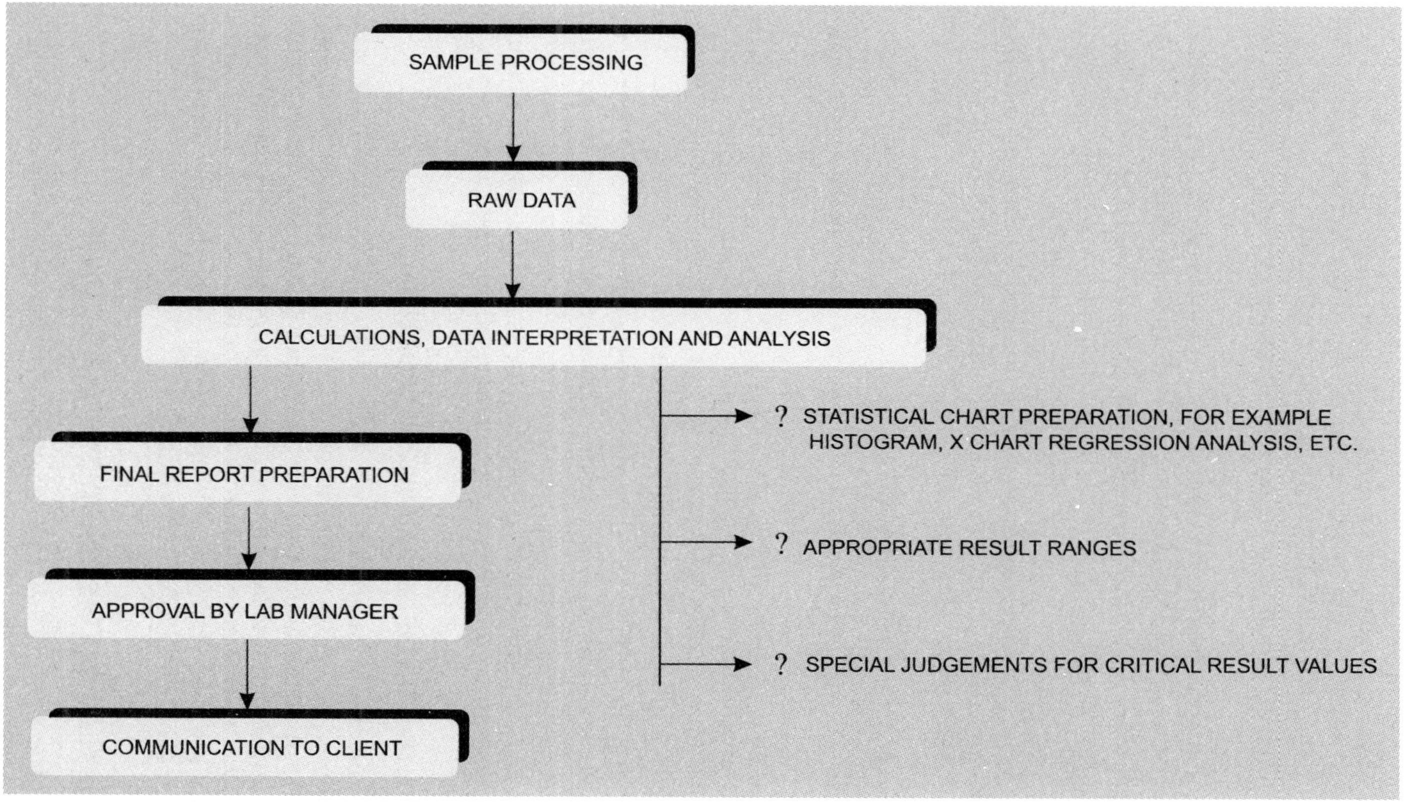

Fig. 6.4: *Flow chart for data calculation and analysis – for special cases, for example: medical diagnoses*

They should be,

- *Understandable* The quality system procedure should be written so clearly that it is understood by the concerned for its proper implementation.
- *Actionable* Appropriate action by test or calibration personnel should be possible.
- *Auditable* The quality system procedure should be properly audited and if required necessary changes should be made to suit the requirements.
- *Mandatory* The quality system procedures should not be optional and resting on the will of the test or calibration personnel. They should be mandatory so that the quality required in test or calibration could be achieved.

Therefore the quality system procedures should be audited by internal auditors and reviewed by laboratory management to meet the internal clients requirements within the laboratory.

A quality system procedure should specifically mention,

What has to be Done The function of the section or division of laboratory should be explained.

Who will do it The responsibilities of test or calibration personnel associated with the section or division should be described briefly.

How it will be Done There should be reference to standard operating procedures or duly validated nonstandard methods or in-house methods.

When it will be Done Time schedule should be prescribed for the start and completion of testing or calibration if necessary. Those concerned with specific procedures may also be mentioned.

What kind of Quality Documentation and Records are to be Maintained Quality documentation needed for the quality system procedures should be given.

6.4 EXTENT OF DOCUMENTATION OF QUALITY SYSTEM PROCEDURES

When the test or calibration personnel involved in test or calibration have long experience and excellence in working there is no necessity to document each and every procedure. But it is quite difficult to answer that which quality system procedure is to be documented and which one is to be left. When no procedure is documented there shall be chaos in the laboratory while documentation of all the procedures shall create too big a volume. Therefore the procedures affecting specifically the quality of test or calibration need only be documented.

6.5 DECIDING WHO SHOULD WRITE THE QUALITY SYSTEM PROCEDURE

Most of the laboratories would feel happy to assign the job of writing the quality system procedures to consultants. The quality system procedure written by the consultant might not necessarily be suitable, and clear to the test or calibration personnel and might create confusion among the laboratory personnel.

The quality system procedure concerning test or calibration laboratories should be written by only those test or calibration personnel who are directly related with these procedures. But this responsibility should be assigned by the quality manager to the section in-charges under his/her direct supervision.

6.5 EXAMPLES OF LABORATORY QUALITY SYSTEM PROCEDURE

For the convenience of the laboratories two examples (Example 6.1 and 6.2) are given here.

EXAMPLE 6.1

LABORATORY QUALITY SYSTEM PROCEDURE (LQSP – 9)

Laboratory's Name: RTLL	QUALITY SYSTEM PROCEDURE	LQSP NO. : 9
	TITLE: Management Review	Revision: 00
		Page: 1/

Purpose To define procedures and to ensure that the quality system is working and technical competence of the laboratory is regularly reviewed.

Scope All laboratory quality system and technical competence elements.

Reference Quality manual
Laboratory quality system procedures

Definitions

Quality Audit An activity carried out by persons independent of the area under review, to establish whether quality system is complied with in the area.

Documentation Management Review Meeting Agenda and Minutes

Procedures

LQSP 9.1 Frequency of Management Review Meeting
Management Review Meeting shall be held at least after six months.

LQSP 9.2 Management Review Meeting Attendees
The meeting shall be chaired by the chief executive of the laboratory, who may nominate another person to attend a particular meeting. The Quality Manager shall attend all meetings and act as meeting secretary. The persons entitled to attend the meeting shall be all regional managers, technical managers, sectional in-charges of the laboratory.

A quorum for a meeting shall be the chairman (or his nominee), the Quality Manager and other persons entitled to attend the meeting.

LQSP 9.3 Agenda for Management Review Meeting

An agenda for each meting shall be as per format no. LQSP 9.3/1 The subject to be covered in "Any other business" shall be determined by CEO or his nominee in consultation with the quality manager before the meeting and included in the written agenda.

The written agenda using format LQSP 9.3/1 shall be circulated by the quality manager three clear days before the date of the meeting to all persons entitled to attend the meeting.

LQSP 9.3/1 Management Review Meeting Agenda

1. Date ____________
   Day ____________
   Time ____________
   Venu ____________
   Chairman ____________
   Secretary ____________
2. Introductory remark by Chairman
3. Composition of the meeting
4. Minutes of the last meeting
5. Points arising from previous meeting
6. Report from the quality manager covering :
   - Results of internal/external quality audit
   - Corrective actions
   - Surveillance visit by accreditation body
   - Changes to quality system documentation carried out since the last meeting
7. Points arising from Sl. No. 6
8. Reports from customer comments and complaints received since the last meeting.
9. Points arising from Sl. No. 8
10. Any other business:
    a) ____________
    b) ____________
    c) ____________
11. Action points arising from the meeting

12. Date of next meeting

LQSP 9.4 Minutes of the Management Review Meeting

The quality manager shall prepare minutes of each meeting, circulate these minutes to all persons entitled to attend the meeting. The minutes shall be signed by the CEO as a true record for the next meeting held.

Approved by	Prepared by	Date of issue

EXAMPLE 6.2

LABORATORY QUALITY SYSTEM PROCEDURE (LQSP –8)

Laboratory's Name: RTLL	QUALITY SYSTEM PROCEDURE	LQSP NO. : 8
	TITLE: Internal Audit	Revision: 00
		Page: 1/

Purpose

1. The aim of internal audit is an attempt to monitor the procedures followed in the laboratory, for the purpose of limiting the scope of investigation when problem arises and also to seek improvement in practice.
2. To train its personnel to perform the assigned task.
3. To establish conformity to regulatory authorities and national or international accreditation bodies.

Scope The internal audit shall be conducted for documented procedures of quality system and related technical procedures followed in the laboratory.

Reference Quality manual
Laboratory quality system procedures

Definitions

Quality Audit : An activity carried out by persons independent of the area under review, to establish whether quality system is complied with in the area.

Documentation: Internal audit schedule form
Internal audit format

Procedures

LQSP 8.1 - *Responsibility of Internal Audit:*

The laboratory quality manager shall identify and assign the responsibility internal audit to well qualified, experienced and trained staff belonging to areas other than the areas to be audited.

LQSP 8.2 – *Internal Audit Schedule:*

LQSP 8.2.1 The internal audit schedule shall cover the quality system and technical areas related to drugs and pharmaceuticals, water, food, general chemicals and microbiology.

LQSP 8.2.1.1 The detailed internal audit schedule shall be followed yearly for quality system documentation including quality manual, SOPs, work instructions and records of personnel training, instrument calibration, subcontracting of tests, complaint redress, data transfer, laboratory consumables purchase, equipment log book, environment monitoring and reference materials related to drugs and pharmaceuticals, water, food, general chemicals and microbiology. The detailed yearly internal audit schedule shall be carried out as highlighted in the LQSP 8/1, 8/1.1, 8/1.2, 8/1.3 (Refer example 6.3–6.6).

LQSP 8.2.2 The laboratory internal audit schedule shall change in case of urgency of external regulatory authority audit or customer complaint.

LQSP 8.3 – *Internal Audit's Frequency:*

The internal audit shall be conducted quarterly. The frequency of internal audit shall be increased or decreased depending on the critical nature of the activity/function.

LQSP 8.4 – *Internal Auditor's Responsibility:*

LQSP 8.4.1 The auditor shall prepare a check list for activity or procedure to be audited. He shall negotiate time with the staff involved in the auditing.

LQSP 8.4.2 The auditor shall report his findings on the prescribed internal audit report format as shown at LQSP 8.2 (Example 6.7). He shall submit the report to the quality manager.

LQSP 8.5 - *Nonconformity compliance and verification:*

LQSP 8.5.1 The quality manager shall issue instructions to staff for taking corrective action for non-conformities observed during the internal audit. (Ref. LQSP 8.3, Example 6.8)

LQSP 8.5.2 The quality manager shall verify the compliance of corrective action taken by the concerned staff against non-conformities. (Ref. LQSP 8.4, Example 6.9)

LQSP 8.5.3 The quality manager shall summarise the internal audit findings and make his recommendation to management for its consideration in the review meeting.

EXAMPLE 6.3

INTERNAL AUDIT SCHEDULE FORM (LQSP 8/1):

NAME OF THE LABORATORY: RTLL

INTERNAL AUDIT SCHEDULE:

PRODUCT OR MATERIAL	ACTIVITY/ FUNCTION	MONTH OF THE YEAR											
		Jan	Feb	Mar	Apr	May	Jun	Jul	Aug	Sep	Oct	Nov	Dec
Drugs and Pharmaceuticals	Quality System Documents and Records												
	Personnel Training												
	Instruments Calibration												
	Laboratory Environment Monitoring												
	Consumable Purchase												
	Samples Handling												
	Test Method/ Internal Calibration Method												
	Reference Materials/ CRM/SRM												
	Complaints Redressel												
	Subcontract of Test on Product/Calibration												
	Internal Quality Techniques Control												
	Effectiveness of Internal Audits												

EXAMPLE 6.4

INTERNAL AUDIT SCHEDULE FORM (LQSP 8/1.1):

NAME OF THE LABORATORY: RTLL

INTERNAL AUDIT SCHEDULE:

PRODUCT OR MATERIAL	ACTIVITY/ FUNCTION	MONTH OF THE YEAR											
		Jan	Feb	Mar	Apr	May	Jun	Jul	Aug	Sep	Oct	Nov	Dec
Food	Records												
	Personnel Training												
	Instruments Calibration												
	Laboratory Environment Monitoring												
	Consumable Purchase												
	Samples Handling												
	Test Method/Internal												
	Calibration Method Reference Materials/ CRM/SRM												
	Complaints Redressel												
	Subcontract of Test on Product/Calibration												
	Internal Quality Control Techniques												
	Effectiveness of Internal Audits												

Example 6.5

INTERNAL AUDIT SCHEDULE FORM (LQSP 8/1.2):

NAME OF THE LABORATORY: RTLL

INTERNAL AUDIT SCHEDULE:

PRODUCT OR MATERIAL	ACTIVITY/ FUNCTION	MONTH OF THE YEAR											
		Jan	Feb	Mar	Apr	May	Jun	Jul	Aug	Sep	Oct	Nov	Dec
Water	Records												
	Personnel Training												
	Instruments Calibration												
	Laboratory Environment Monitoring												
	Consumable Purchase												
	Samples Handling												
	Test Method/Internal Calibration Method												
	Reference Materials/ CRM/SRM												
	Complaints Redressel												
	Subcontract of Test on Product/Calibration												
	Internal Quality Control Techniques												
	Effectiveness of Internal Audits												

EXAMPLE 6.6

INTERNAL AUDIT SCHEDULE FORM (LQSP 8/1.3):

NAME OF THE LABORATORY: RTLL

INTERNAL AUDIT SCHEDULE:

PRODUCT OR MATERIAL	ACTIVITY/ FUNCTION	MONTH OF THE YEAR											
		Jan	Feb	Mar	Apr	May	Jun	Jul	Aug	Sep	Oct	Nov	Dec
General Chemicals	Records												
	Personnel Training												
	Instruments Calibration												
	Laboratory Environment Monitoring												
	Consumable Purchase												
	Samples Handling												
	Test Method/Internal Calibration Method												
	Reference Materials/ CRM/SRM												
	Complaints Redressel												
	Subcontract of Test on Product/Calibration												
	Internal Quality Control Techniques												
	Effectiveness of Internal Audits												

EXAMPLE 6.7

INTERNAL AUDIT REPORT FORMAT (LQSP 8/8.2)

NAME OF THE LABORATORY:

NAME OF THE AUDITOR: IARF NO.:

AREA UNDER INTERNAL AUDIT:

ACTIVITY/FUNCTION AUDITED:

NONCONFORMITY OBSERVED:

SERIOUSNESS OF THE NONCONFORMITY:

RECOMMENDATION:

SIGNATURE OF THE AUDITOR: DATE:

QUALITY MANAGER:

APPROVED BY:	PREPARED BY:	DATE OF ISSUE:

EXAMPLE 6.8

CORRECTIVE ACTION FORM (LQSP 8/8.3)

(RESPONSIBILITY ASSIGNED TO STAFF BY QUALITY MANAGER)

NAME OF STAFF:

AREA UNDER WHICH NONCONFORMITY IS OBSERVED:

DATE OF INTERNAL AUDIT DONE:

NAME OF OFFICER RECTIFYING NONCONFORMITY:

ACTION TAKEN FOR COMPLIANCE:

SIGNATURE OF STAFF: DATE:

NONCONFORMITY COMPLIANCE REPORTED TO QUALITY MANAGER ON:

(QUALITY MANAGER)

APPROVED BY:	PREPARED BY:	DATE OF ISSUE:

EXAMPLE 6.9

NONCONFORMITY COMPLIANCE VERIFICATION FORM (LQSP 8/8.4)

VERIFICATION OF CONFORMITY:

SIGNATURE OF QUALITY MANAGER:

DATE:

APPROVED BY:	PREPARED BY:	DATE OF ISSUE:

7

Standard Operating Procedures and Laboratory Work Instructions

7.1 INTRODUCTION

It is of utmost importance to understand what is a standard operating procedure. The Standard Operating Procedures (SOPs) are "well defined working instructions for an operating procedure whose course is clearly documented. The instructions must be followed as accurately as possible to ensure the comparability of the results". The Standard Operating Procedures are third level documentation of laboratory quality system which are required to elaborate a specific test or calibration procedure, or method, equipment's maintenance or cleaning procedure being followed in the laboratory to achieve the correct test or calibration results.

As the name implies the Standard Operating Procedures are brief, concise testing, calibration, maintenance or cleaning methods formulated by the laboratory for day to day in-house use which has reference to products, specifications, separate method standards, manufacturer equipment maintenance manual, national or international pharmacopoeias, text books or technical journals of repute.

The Standard Operating Procedures as third level documentation are used to guide the test, calibration, equipment/instrument maintenance or cleaning personnel to obtain the quality in test or calibration. Thus SOPs can be categorized as follows:

- Testing SOPs
- Calibration SOPs
- Equipment/Instrument Maintenance SOPs
- Cleaning SOPs
- Inspection SOPs

The laboratory must document the Standard Operating Procedures in an appropriate manner as unwritten instruction may not be remembered by the test, calibration and maintenance personnel for their implementation in the laboratory.

7.2 NECESSITY OF STANDARD OPERATING PROCEDURES

The SOPs are essential to implement a valid test or calibration method, equipment maintenance procedure, cleaning or inspection procedure. The Standard Operating Procedures of system suitability test are required to prove whether the measurement system is suitable for planned measurement or determination while ensuring compliance with defined tolerances. Suitable operating procedures can be used to ensure the system suitability or reliability of the complete measurement system. Thus on establishing that the system suitability is successfully ensured, the routine operation can be started. A check list based on the Standard Operating Procedure must be made at regular intervals to see whether the particular measurement performance of the equipment/ instrument is still within the tolerances as originally specified.

7.3 DEVELOPING THE STANDARD OPERATING PROCEDURES

In order to develop Standard Operating Procedures it is essential that the one who develops it must be familiar with the standard being practiced for such type of testing, calibration, maintenance, cleaning or inspection. The personnel while developing the Standard Operating Procedures should give priority to the following:

- SOPs must comply to the established laboratory requirement for testing or calibration to achieve the reliable results.
- The SOP should contain all successive steps of the activities for which it is made.
- The participation of test or calibration personnel in development of SOPs.
- Contents of the SOP and the administrative matters should be decided.
- Data collection and evaluation.

The Standard Operating Procedures must have uniformity in their content and to maintain the same a format should be developed by the concerned laboratory. The format should have at least the following (Fig. 7.1):

STANDARD OPERATING PROCEDURES	FORMAT
Cover - Administrative aspects, technical requirements, references of current specifications, standards, textbooks, etc. **Types-** SOPs for testing, calibration in equipments/instruments, maintenance, cleaning, inspection, etc.	Numbering, title, name of test/calibration equipment, nature of materials needed, description of documentation, data processing and evaluation, documents and samples to be stored, approval and authorization, reference.

Fig. 7.1: *Standard Operating Procedures —features and format contents*

Name of laboratory: RTLL	STANDARD OPERATING PROCEDURE	SOP NO.:
	TITLE: Standard Operating Procedures formulation	Revision: Page:

1. SOP numbering: The SOP developed should be given a unique number for identification and each page be given numbers (1 to n).
2. Title: There should be a title for the SOP.
3. Name of test or calibration equipment: The SOP should have appropriate information about the testing or calibrating instruments. The SOP should mention the range along with accuracy of the test or calibration equipment.
4. Nature of Material needed: The SOP should possess information regarding various material such as reagent, thermometers, indicators, mandrill and other items required for testing or calibration.
5. Description of test or calibration steps: The SOP, for appropriate understanding, should consist of various steps involved in testing or calibration of items.
6. Description of documentation: The documentation for SOP should be developed and have references to internal or external documentation.
7. Data processing and evaluation: The SOP here highlights the procedure of calculation to arrive on test or calibration results. It should also enumerate the evaluation procedure for correctness of data.
8. Documents and sample to be stored : The SOP should have information of documents, and samples to be retained for further action.
9. Approval and authorization: The SOP should be duly approved and authorized to persons by competent higher authority.
10. References: The SOP must have reference of the standard, specification or valid technical journal or books from where the test or calibration procedure or methods are drawn.

Approved by	Prepared by	Date of Issue

7.4 SCOPE OF STANDARD OPERATING PROCEDURES

The SOP plays an important role in documentation required by the relevant Quality Standard. The Standard Operating Procedure is always matched with the method and the condition on the site. In practice the Standard Operating Procedure formulated by the user is read and followed much more attentively by the fellow employee than the one produced by an anonymous authority. The following essential parameters should be covered in each Standard Operating Procedure (Fig. 7.1) :

a. SOP should cover the administrative matters, like
   - Use of SOP format
   - Name of equipment and serial number
   - Date of SOP produced
   - Storage identification
   - Page numbering
   - Title
   - Date of implementation
   - Information on revisions
   - Specification of departments responsible for implementation
   - Date of signature, authors, checkers, persons responsible for authorization
   - Distribution

b. SOP should cover the technical requirements, like
   - Test or calibration material
   - Sampling procedure
   - Sample preparation
   - Successive steps of test or calibration
   - Data recording
   - Calculation procedure
   - Documentation
   - Equipment range and accuracy details
   - Test or calibration reference condition
   - Use of CRM/SRM for standardization

c. SOP should have references, like those of current specification, standard, text book, pharmacopoeia, or from where it is abstracted

7.5 RESPONSIBILITY FOR DEVELOPING STANDARD OPERATING PROCEDURES

The development of Standard Operating Procedure is an important task before the laboratories. Thus this type of job can not be assigned to the persons who do not have experience test or calibration. The laboratories having sufficient staff with appropriate experience must assign this responsibility to section incharge responsible for performance of test or calibration. Therefore, the laboratory should assign the responsibility to the persons having comprehensive knowledge of method specification, standard text book, technical journal, pharmacopoeia etc. being followed for respective test or calibration method/procedure.

These persons should have detailed knowledge of the equipment/instrument parameter of the required accuracy and their functions to be used for determining the test or calibration results. The persons should be acquainted with data collection, calculation and evaluation.

7.6 APPROVAL, ISSUE AND CONTROL OF SOPs

The Standard Operating Procedure which is formulated must have approval of the competent personnel as described in the Quality Manual of the laboratory. In general it has approval of the technical manager, technical director or as the case may be, but after appropriate checks.

The date of issue for implementation in the respective departments is also of importance as these departments strictly comply to the requirements of the SOP.

The SOP so approved should be marked as "controlled" while it is put in use by the respective department, section or division of the laboratory. The SOP may bear a mark with appropriate symbol or stamped as "CONTROLLED".

7.7 MAINTENANCE OF SOPs

The maintenance of SOP can be ensured through validation of the methods, or procedures. The laboratory should have a system of continuous assessment of the method/procedure. If the laboratory makes any changes in successive steps required to arrive at a result then the SOP becomes a Non- Standard Operating Procedure. This type of procedure must be established by the laboratory through validation, alternate calculation etc. to make them appropriate SOP.

The laboratory should develop a practice of maintenance of SOP through validation whenever it is found that the results are not reliable.

7.7.1 Dynamic Management of Information Generated at Various Stages of a Standard Operating Procedure

Either quality manager or a technical manager should be assigned the task of keeping track of information generated at various stages of a SOP and recording of that information. This should be aimed at dynamic reutilization of the accumulated information towards quality assurance to clients. Users may specially refer to the elucidative Fig. 7.2 given here as an example of accumulation of information at various stages of sample handling.

7.8 THE EXTENT OF SOP DOCUMENTATION

The SOP can be made for inspection, testing, calibration, cleanliness or equipment/instrument maintenance. But the foremost question is whether a laboratory should develop Standard Operating Procedures for each and every type of standard available with the laboratory?

If this is so, it will take years to make SOP for each and every test or calibration. Therefore it should not be made mandatory. The SOP should be made for those tests or calibrations which are critical in nature or may cause injury to humans or affect the environment. The laboratory should also make Standard Operating Procedures for analysis of hazardous materials or substances. For example the laboratories associated with testing of biological, microbiological, clinical, hazardous chemicals should develop SOPs. The laboratories associated with testing of electrical, mechanical or electronics items need not necessarily spend their time in developing SOP since reference specifications, standards are sufficient in such cases.

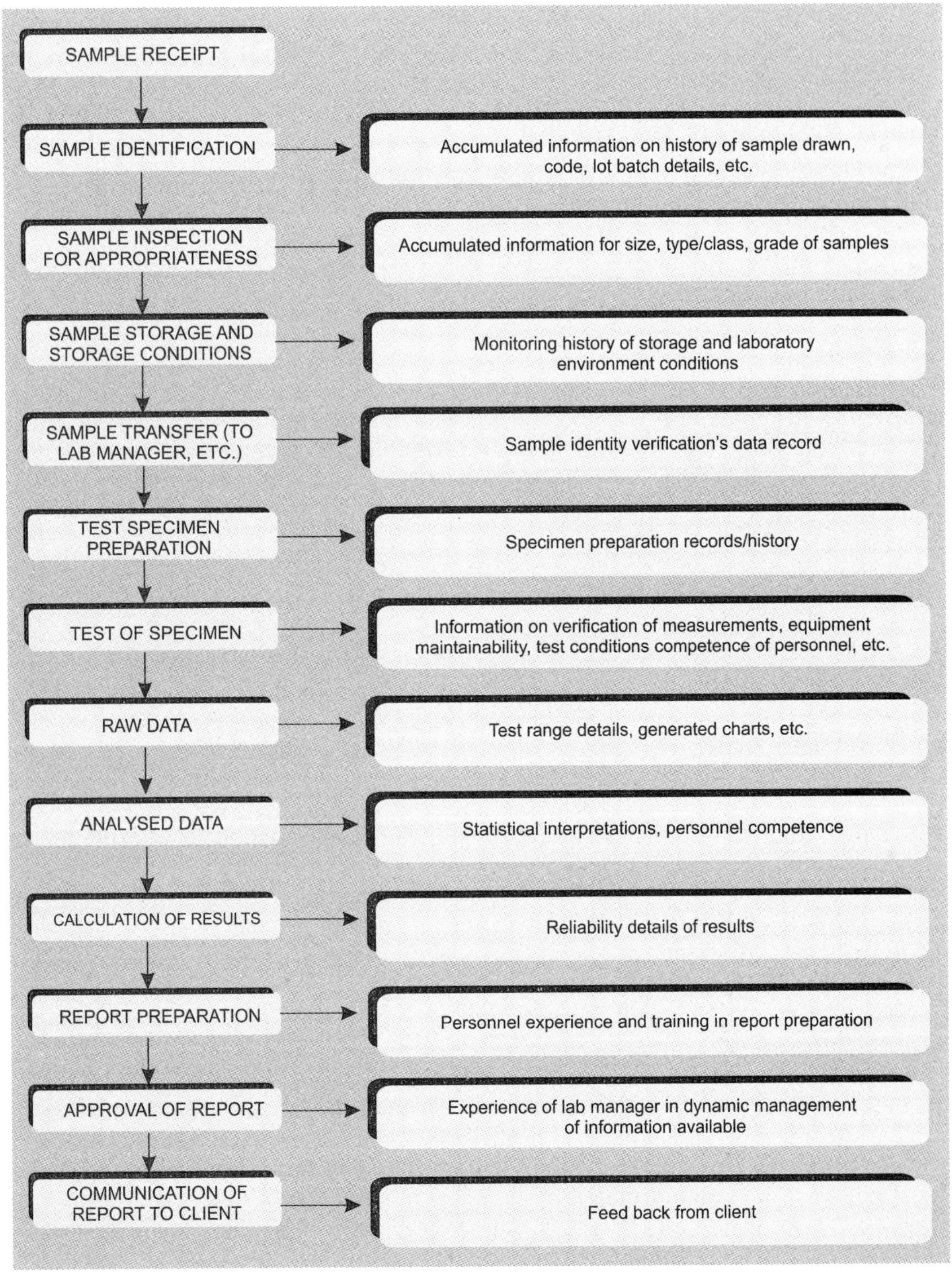

Fig. 7.2: *Information generation at various stages of sample handling*

A laboratory which makes certain changes, for example in some chemical concentration needed under the relevant SOP to arrive at the requisite requirement to standardize the procedure, must also document the validation of SOP.

7.9 EXAMPLES OF STANDARD OPERATING PROCEDURES

The following examples (7.1 and 7.2) may be used by the laboratories for developing the Standard Operating Procedures.

EXAMPLE 7.1

Name of laboratory:RTLL	STANDARD OPERATING PROCEDURE	SOP No. : 01
	TITLE: CLEANING LABORATORY APPARATUS (RELATED TO TRACE METAL ANALYSIS)	Revision : 00 Page: 1/

1. The procedure details the steps for cleaning laboratory apparatus, sample containers and High Density Polyethylene (HDPE) and Low Density Polyethylene sampling equipments used for trace metal sampling and analyses.
2. Removal of organic residues and dust shall be done in a soap solution, followed by several rounds of rinsing with metal free water.
3. Acid bath series :
   (i) Baths of Nitric Acid (Conc.) reagent grade and Hydrochloric Acid (Conc.) reagent grade shall be used for cleaning HDPE and LDPE equipments coupled with rinsing with metal free water before and after each step. Then the equipment shall be stored in 1% Hydrochloric Acid.
   (ii) Nitric Acid (Conc.) baths shall be used twice for cleaning PTFE (Poly tetrafluoroethylene) equipments coupled with rinsing with metal free water before and after each step. Then the equipment shall be stored in 1% Hydrochloric Acid.
   (iii) If necessary, the acid baths shall be heated before use.
4. The apparatus shall be rinsed thrice in de-ionised water and dried for one hour at 80° C in oven.
5. The cleaned laboratory apparatus shall be stored in double zipped bags and in dust free, metal contamination free spaces/racks.

Description of documentation: Quality Manual
SOP Manual

Approved by	Prepared by	Date of Issue

EXAMPLE 7.2

Name of laboratory:RTLL	STANDARD OPERATING PROCEDURE	SOP No. : 02
	TITLE: DOCUMENTATION OF NOTEBOOKS, LOGBOOKS	Revision : 00 Page:1/1

1. The procedure shall be observed for all the procedures operated in the laboratory.
2. The procedure is applicable to all the run logs for instruments, logbooks for instrument maintenance, digestions, and miscellaneous documentation (like oven and refrigerator temperature monitoring), analyst's notebooks for method development, problem solving, trouble shooting
3. All notebooks shall be maintained as primary analytical record and as controlled copies. It shall be signed by the notebook holder and his non-analysing colleague at the end of the day.
4. All notebooks are subject to monthly review by internal peers who shall cover at least 20% of all the entries.
5. All the logbooks, analytical and miscellaneous, shall be signed by the persons conducting the procedures and shall be used for monthly peer review for at least 20% of the entries
6. All the staff are provided with a copy of this standard operating procedure so as to ensure compliance.

Description of documentation: Quality Manual
S O P Manual

Approved by	Prepared by	Date of Issue

7.10 INTRODUCTION TO LABORATORY WORK INSTRUCTIONS

Work instruction is a generic term which can be used for initiating action to commence an activity. There are various activities in the laboratory which should be documented as laboratory work instructions by the laboratory testing or calibration supervisor to guide the fellow staff for efficient and appropriate implementation of an activity. These laboratory work instructions may include various activities. Some of them are as follows :

- Filling of test request by client
- Receipt sample handling by the laboratory
- Sample preparation for test or calibration
- Equipment operation

- Standard solution preparation and retention
- House keeping
- Test report dispatch
- Complaint filing by the clients
- Safety during the test
- Hazardous substances handling
- Use of reference materials
- Storing of Certified Reference Materials
- Restructured areas instructions

The laboratory work instructions may be in several forms :

- Verbal
- Written
- Sample drawing
- Computer menu options for calculation

It is really difficult to follow the verbal laboratory work instructions given to the test or calibration personnel. Therefore laboratories should avoid such practice while developing sound, effective quality systems.

7.11 SCOPE OF LABORATORY WORK INSTRUCTIONS

The laboratory work instructions should be developed in such a way that the required instructions are covered in a brief manner. The brief subject matter should be clearly understood by the concerned test or calibration personnel involved in administration of the same. The basic objective of laboratory work instructions is to familiarize the personnel with general requisites associated with a sound laboratory quality system. For example the personnel associated with the receipt of the test or calibration items should be aware of what is to be covered in the TEST or CALIBRATION REQUEST FORM given to the client by the laboratory at the time of handing over the sample. The person in question should ask the client to fill up the TEST REQUEST FORM before he leaves the premises of the laboratory.

The contents of laboratory work instructions should cover the following :

- Title
- Scope
- Purpose
- Activity subject matter
- Assigned responsibility
- Records to maintain
- Authority to issue
- Control

The laboratories should not develop work instructions for each and every activity as that would lead to a too large number of laboratory work instructions.

7.12 EXAMPLES OF LABORATORY WORK INSTRUCTIONS

EXAMPLE 7.3

TEST REQUEST FORM

Name of Laboratory : RTLL	LABORATORY WORK	LABORATORY WORK INSTRUCTIONS : 12
	TITLE: Test Request Form	Revision: 00 Page 1/1

Scope: This sample Test Request Form (TRF) shall be used by the laboratory for the test or calibration samples received from the clients.

Purpose: The TRF is to be filled in by the client for confirming the nature of the tests to be conducted on the sample by the test laboratory.

Activity Subject Matter:

- Client should mention the details of the sample (sample size)
- Client should mention the nature of tests to be conducted on the sample.
- Client should mention current specification against which tests are to be done.
- Client should mention reference conditions of tests if specific.
- Client should mention test result delivery conditions.

Assigned Responsibility:
This responsibility is assigned to Sh. R.K. Palival, asst. clerk. In his absence it shall be looked after by the concerned supervisor of sample receipt section.

Records to be maintained:
RTLL shall maintain the records of TRF and retain the same for a period of six months.

Authority to issue:
Laboratory Quality Manager is authorized to issue laboratory work instructions.

Control:
The laboratory work instructions will be controlled through a unique numbering system and any change in the subject matter shall be incorporated and new laboratory work instruction shall be issued after due approval of the laboratory quality manager.

Approved by	Prepared by	Date of Issue

EXAMPLE 7.4

TEST REQUEST FORM

Name of Laboratory : RTLL	LABORATORY WORK INSTRUCTIONS	LABORATORY WORK INSTRUCTIONS : 13
	TITLE: Laboratory Housekeeping Form	Revision: 00 Page 1/1

Scope: Laboratory house keeping shall be applicable to all testing laboratories associated with RTLL.

Purpose: Laboratory house keeping is required to up keep the appropriate levels cleanliness through stacking of reagents, samples, reference materials, appropriate electrical wiring, discrimination of hazardous test areas, safety provision, approach road, glass ware and records.

Activity Subject Matter :

- The floor of the laboratory should be kept clean.
- All instruments, equipments should be cleaned weekly.
- All samples should be labeled and kept under controlled conditions.
- Doors, windows, and walls should have appropriate paints.
- Laboratory should be free from acid fumes and appropriate level of fresh air should be maintained.
- All reports, records and quality documents should be kept in almirahs or cupboards in archives.
- Sign boards should be used for guidance of the customer's entry to restricted areas, where hazardous samples are tested.
- Urinals and lavatory should be kept clean.
  Laboratory should have arrangements for integrated lights.
- All instruments, either in repair or unused, should have labeling.
- Laboratory should have concealed electrical wiring, and change over switch or step down transformer should be kept outside the laboratory.
- Laboratory should have dust controller for sophisticated instrumentation.
- All safety equipments should be checked once in a month.
- All reference materials should be labeled and kept properly.
- Laboratory should have good approach roads.

Assigned Responsibility:

This responsibility is assigned to deputy quality manager. In his absence it shall be looked after by the concerned supervisor of each testing laboratory.

Records to be maintained:

RTLL shall maintain the records of house keeping and retain the same for a period of six months.

Authority to issue:

Laboratory Quality Manager is authorized to issue laboratory work instructions.

Control:

The laboratory work instructions will be controlled through a unique numbering system. Any change in the subject matter shall be incorporated and new laboratory work instruction issued after due approval of laboratory quality manager.

Approved by	Prepared by	Date of Issue

8

Quality Documents

8.1 INTRODUCTION

Every system for its effective operation requires documentation of essential activities related to it because with out a written document the laboratory personnel will face tremendous difficulties in achieving the objectives mentioned in the quality policy. Similarly the laboratory accreditation requires quality documents which include in general — forms, formats, records or reports. The most commonly used quality documents in a number of laboratories are forms, formats, reports and records detailed as follows :

Forms

- Store receipt form
- Sample test request form
- Sample handling form
- Test raw data form
- Material requisition form
- Clients complaint form
- Amendment form
- Document distribution form

Formats

- Calibration report format
- Test report format
- Internal audit report format
- Nonconformity report format

- Internal audit plan format
- Conformity report format

Reports

- Equipment preventive maintenance report
- Equipment maintenance report
- Internal calibration report
- Test report
- Client complaint report
- Management review report

Records

- Sample receipt records
- Test or calibration raw data record
- Preventive maintenance record
- Maintenance record
- Calibration record
- Test record
- Internal audit record
- Management review record
- Test Subcontracting record
- Complaint record
- Equipment record/log book
- Consumable inspection record
- Method validation record
- Laboratory environment monitoring record
- Personnel record
- Vendors record

Test or calibration laboratories should maintain such type of forms, formats, reports and records for understanding and efficient implementation of quality documentation to achieve the objective.

The laboratory test or calibration personnel should be clear about the various terms or words used in these quality documents. These quality documents should be legible, accessible and stored under appropriate secured conditions. These quality records should be available as and when required and retained for a period of three years and disposed off in accordance with documented procedure.

8.2 NECESSITY OF FORMS OR FORMATS

The use of forms and formats in test or calibration laboratories is essential to simplify and to standardize the various day to day activities related to test or calibration of internal or external samples. The use of SAMPLE TEST REQUEST FORMS helps the clients in detailing the nature of test to be conducted by the concerned laboratory. The client who does not know the nature of test to be conducted on the sample is helped by the laboratory to tell her competence in the area of testing for such item or sample.

A Sample Test Request Form is given here for the sake of example (Example 8.1):

EXAMPLE 8.1

RAJSHREE TEST LABORATORY LIMITED

(New Delhi)

Test Request Form

TRF No.: Date:

Name of Client :

Client Address :

Phone: Fax:

Nature of Sample received :

Condition of Sample:

Sample's quantity :

Client code (if any) :

Test required by the Client :

Sample No.	Nature of Test	Method Specification No.

Any other information:

Signature of Client
Date:

Signature of Sample Receipt Officer
RTLL
Date:

In the same way various formats developed by the test or calibration laboratories will be useful in standardizing and maintaining uniformity in availability of technical information needed to arrive on decisions for further improvement in the laboratory quality system.

8.3 SCOPE OF TEST REPORT

The laboratory may be having a test report format and using the same for a long period but it is important for laboratory to check whether this test report complies to the requirement of an accreditation criteria or standard on which the accreditation criteria is based. The test report in general should cover at the minimum the following.

1. Name of the test laboratory issuing test report
2. Test report number and date of issue
3. Client's name and address
4. Sample code used by test laboratory
5. Sample receipt date
6. Sample testing date
7. Test reference condition
8. Test method specification
9. Nature of test conducted on sample
10. Test values obtained and corresponding values as stipulated in specification
11. Status of test equipment calibration
12. Legal statement for non appearance in litigation cases by the test laboratory
13. Signature of personnel checking and issuing test report
14. Any other requirement of accreditation standard

8.4 WHAT TO COVER IN A CALIBRATION REPORT

The content of calibration report received by any test or calibration laboratory are of much importance as it establishes the reliability of calibration data generated by the laboratories. The calibration report should contain at the minimum the following.

1. Name of the calibration laboratory issuing the calibration report
2. Calibration report number and date of issue
3. Client's name and address
4. Client's equipment number
5. Equipment receipt date
6. Calibration date
7. Calibration reference conditions
8. Calibration method specification number
9. Nature of range of measurements conducted on calibration equipment/ instrument

10. Calibration values obtained and corresponding values indicated by the calibration instrument
11. Uncertainty of measurement
12. Confidence limit
13. Legal statement for non appearance in litigation cases by the laboratory
14. Signature of personnel checking and issuing calibration reports
15. Any other requirement of accreditation standard

The calibration report should establish the traceability chain and artifact number by which the equipment is calibrated. If calibration report consists of a single reading for a particular measurement then it is not covering the requirement of reproducibility. If necessary, the calculation of uncertainty of measurement should be attached with the calibration report.

8.5 SIGNATORY OF TEST OR CALIBRATION REPORT

The test or calibration laboratories in general should assign this responsibility to the persons having technical knowledge and experience in the appropriate areas of test or calibration. Some times it is observed that the Managing Director who does not have the particular qualification and experience, is signing the test or calibration report. The laboratory management should employ personnel from appropriate areas of test or calibration so that wrong test or calibration report does not reach the hands of clients and damage to the reputation of the laboratory could be avoided.

8.6 APPROVING AUTHORITY OF FORMS OR FORMATS

The forms and formats, which are very much useful in simplifying the day to day work in the laboratory, should not only be carefully prepared but approved by the quality manager after detailed discussions with the supervisor of the concerned area of test or calibration.

Any change in forms and formats should be informed to the concerned user and a record of such changes should be maintained by the authorized personnel.

PART 3

Writing a Laboratory Quality Manual

9

Quality Manual and its Purpose

9.1 QUALITY MANUAL

The most time consuming and sometimes cumbersome task for the laboratory, before the application is sent to the accreditation body, is to prepare the Quality Manual. The Quality Manual should define the procedures to be adopted so as to ensure that the laboratory operations comply with accreditation requirements as given in a national regulation or standard.

The Quality Manual is a key document, therefore it should be an operational document which accurately reflects the activities carried out in the laboratory rather than a document simply produced for the purpose of assessment. The manual must be authorized by the head of the laboratory and there should be a procedure for ensuring that it is kept up-to-date and reviewed periodically.

The laboratory quality manual should define in detail the scope of accreditation and terms of reference of senior technical personnel. It should also contain organizational structure, normally in the form of a chart, as well as interrelationship of management, technical operation support services and quality assurance.

The Quality Manual should set out or contain reference to detailed operating procedures covering all the requirements of accreditation as laid down in the national regulation or standard. Provided that the manual contains clear identifying references, it needs not contain every detail of the laboratory's accredited activities.

The large scale laboratories may prefer to prepare separate documents covering for example calibration, sample handling, equipment maintenance operating procedures or staff training. On the other hand small laboratories often find it most convenient to include all the operating procedures in the Quality Manual.

In the case of the companies holding certificate for their quality system according to ISO 9001/9002, their testing laboratories may refer to the main Quality Manual of the company or a number of general quality assurance requirements for example quality policy, quality management, quality audit and staff training.

In case of a principal laboratory which has a number of sister laboratories at different locations in the country, all the sister laboratories should have the Quality Manual for each individual laboratory. The necessity to prepare a separate Quality Manual by the sister laboratory is owing to difference in the scope of accreditation, facilities, organization of quality management, etc.

9.2 PURPOSE OF QUALITY MANUAL

The Quality Manual can be used by the laboratories for various purposes which are given as follows:

1. To meet the specified requirements of national regulation of standards based on ISO/IEC Guide 25:1990 and latest standard of laboratory accreditation ISO 17025:1999 for establishing the competence or the accreditation of the laboratories.
2. To communicate quality policy and objectives of the laboratory to its personnel or customers.
3. To provide appropriate description of policies or procedure, effective implementation and maintenance of the laboratory quality systems.
4. To maintain continuity and consistency in operation of laboratory quality system in the face of any changes in the laboratory organization.
5. To ensure orderliness in operation by giving clear description of quality assurance practices.
6. To train the laboratory test or calibration personnel on quality system as well as technical competence requirements.
7. To guide the testing subcontractors to comply with the requirements of laboratory accreditation prior to the contract.
8. To provide base for internal and external audit of quality system and technical competence performance of laboratory.
9. To satisfy and convince the customer regarding capability and technical competence of the laboratory.
10. Quality Manual can be used as a business tool to secure international business.

9.3 STRUCTURE OF QUALITY MANUAL

There is no well defined form or style in which the laboratory Quality Manual is to be presented but there can be a format which can be adopted to formulate a laboratory Quality Manual. The format for structure of Quality Manual to be used by the test or calibration laboratories should have at least the laboratory title, the chapter number, revision number, page number, and chapter title on each page. The structure of laboratory quality manual should include the following :

- Company Title
- Laboratory title
- Manual's table of content
- Scope of Quality Manual

- Introductory pages for the laboratory and the company
- Manual Issue number, date of issue
- Amendment status with record
- Authority to issue Quality Manual and respective amendments
- Glossary of standard terms used in Quality Manual
- Distribution list
- Laboratory quality policy and objectives
- Organization for laboratory quality assurance
- Reference of standard operating procedures
- Reference of quality procedures
- Description of laboratory quality system elements
- Description of elements of technical competence for laboratory

Title of the Company/laboratory The Quality Manual should have the name of the company to which the laboratory belongs or if independent it should have its own title accordingly.

Manual's Table of Contents The table of contents of the laboratory Quality Manual should reflect the title of chapters and the easiest method of tracing them in the manual.

Scope of Quality Manual The Quality Manual should reflect the scope of areas of accreditation for which the laboratory has submitted its application to a national or international accreditation body.

Introductory Pages for the Laboratory and Company The introductory pages of the Quality Manual should describe in brief the profile of the company to which the laboratory belongs. It should mention the location of the laboratory and its relation with the concerned company.

Manual Issue Number, Date of Issue and Amendment Status The laboratory Quality Manual should have its issue number, the date of issue and appropriate status of amendment in the amendment sheet. The status of amendment should mention the latest revision number and date for each chapter, duly signed by the quality manager.

Authority to Issue Quality Manual and Respective Amendments The manual should describe the procedure and authority to issue, amend, revise and distribute its controlled copies to the concerned section's head.

Glossary of Standard Terms used in the Quality Manual The Quality Manual should describe the interpretation of terms or definitions used in the Quality Manual for the understanding of users.

Distribution List The distribution list should also cover the name of the accreditation body and updated controlled copy of the Quality Manual should be sent to the national accreditation body.

Laboratory Quality Policy and Objectives The Quality Manual should describe the Quality Policy of the laboratory. If the laboratory is the part of a company, it should redefine its laboratory quality policy according to the requirements of the laboratory accreditation of the national or international standard. The laboratory quality policy should not be contradictory to the company's quality policy.

Organization for Laboratory's Quality Assurance The Quality Manual should consist of the operative organization chart of the personnel involved in the testing or calibration laboratory. The job description of the individual persons should be defined along with their interrelations with other sections in the laboratory or departments in the company. The Quality Manual should cover the reference of various techniques of laboratory quality assurance such as repeat analysis, replicate analysis, SQC (Statistical Quality Control) techniques, inter/intra laboratory comparison.

Reference of Standard Operating Procedures The Quality Manual should describe the reference of Standard Operating Procedures used for test or calibration of item or samples. If the laboratory in general is using test or calibration methods taken from national or international specifications, there is no necessity to provide the reference of specifications in the Quality Manual but a paragraph, mentioning that the laboratory follows standard test or calibration method from specifications, should only be mentioned. If the test or calibration method is taken from reputed journals or text books then a Standard Operating Procedure should be formulated by the laboratories and should be referred in the manual.

10

Contents of the Laboratory Quality Manual

10.1 CONTENTS OF QUALITY MANUAL

The Quality Manual specifically and precisely defines the quality related tasks to be performed by the various sections of the laboratory to achieve the objectives as described in the laboratory quality policy.

For the contents of a laboratory Quality Manual there is no fixed rule or fixed structure in any international standard. The contents of the laboratory quality Manual basically depend on the organization with which the laboratory is associated and the various areas of test or calibration being taken up by the laboratory for accreditation. The Quality Manual in general describes the elements of the laboratory quality system, technical competence, reference to quality procedures and standard operating procedures.

The contents of the Quality Manual do not describe the technical details of test or calibration performed or methods of use of reference materials, certified material or secondary reference material by the laboratory. Therefore it can be given to customers after specifying them as controlled or uncontrolled copies.

The ISO/IEC Guide 25:1990 under clause 5.2 has described minimum contents of the Laboratory Quality Manual which are as follows:

1. Quality Policy statement, objective and commitment
2. Organization and management structure of the laboratory, relation to parent organization and organization chart
3. Interrelation between management, technical operation, support service and quality system.
4. Document control and maintenance procedures
5. Job description of key staff
6. Identification of approved signatories

7. Laboratory procedure to achieve traceability of measurements
8. Laboratory's scope of test or calibration
9. Review of facilities for commencing new work
10. Procedures for handling of test or calibration item
11. Reference to equipment and reference measurement standards
12. Reference to procedures for calibration, verification and maintenance of equipments
13. Reference to inter-laboratory comparison, proficiency testing programme, reference material and internal quality control schemes
14. Procedures for feedback and corrective action for discrepancies observed in testing or departure from documented policies and procedures
15. Laboratory management arrangement for permitting exceptions of departure from the documented policies and procedures or standard specifications
16. Procedures for dealing with the complaints
17. Procedures for protecting confidentiality and proprietary rights
18. Procedure for audit and review

The minimum contents as described under the clause 5.2 of ISO/IEC Guide 25:1990 do not include test or calibration personnel training, laboratory's environment, its monitoring and accommodation, calibration policy and schedules, test or calibration method, validation of methods, sampling procedures, test or calibration certificates, subcontracting of test or calibration and records retention.

Thus the contents of laboratory quality manual should describe the each and every element of quality system and technical competence as specified in the accreditation criteria or national or international standards for laboratory accreditation.

The content of Quality Manual should also describe the procedures of reaffirmation, review, amendment, approval and issue of quality documentation.

10.2 ORGANIZATION STRUCTURE OF THE LABORATORY

The laboratory should describe its operational organizational structure through block diagrams (Fig. 10.1). If the laboratory is independent then the organizational charts not only reflect its hierarchy but also the operational organization charts and their relation with the various types of laboratories operating from the same premises.

The laboratories which are a part of a company should show through block diagrams in their organizational charts the relation of the concerned laboratory with the parent company and personnel of the other related departments.

The test or calibration laboratories which are having sister concerns or subsidiary laboratories in different parts of the country should show operational organizational chart of subsidiary laboratory and its relation with the parent laboratory through block diagram in their Quality Manual.

The operational organizational chart should clearly show the access of quality manager to the top management.

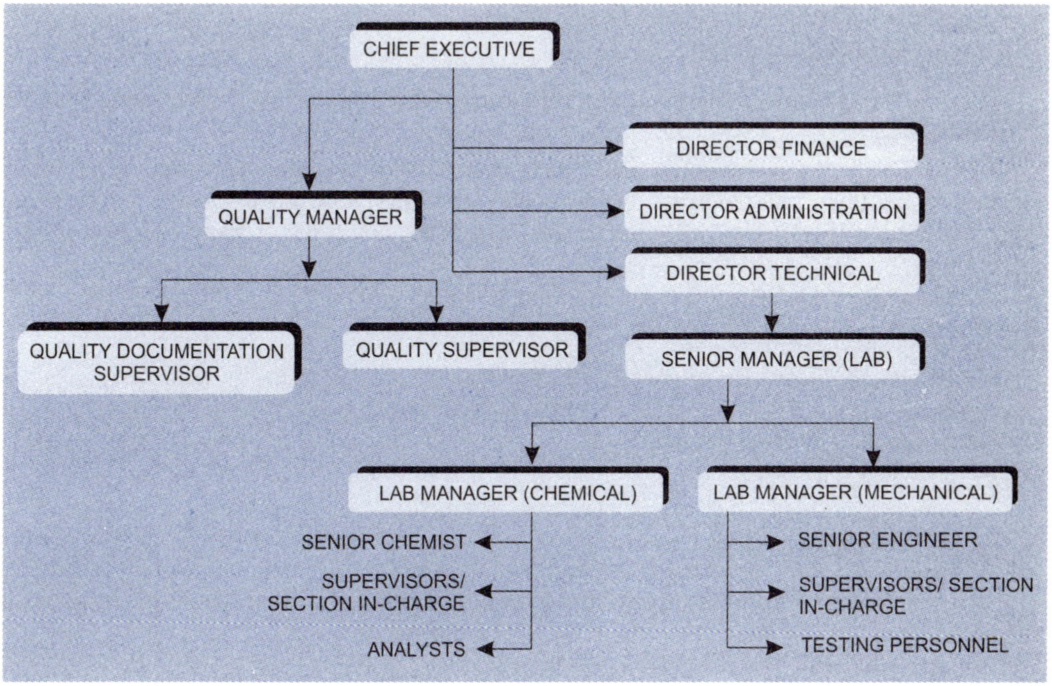

Fig. 10.1: *Operational organization chart of laboratory*

The section heads and the subordinates should also be shown in case the laboratory is dealing with different areas of testing or calibration.

The operating organization chart should reflect the position of the technical manager and supervisors of various sections of the laboratory. The operational organization chart of the small laboratory can show the position of quality manager cum technical manager and other supervisors.

10.3 ELEMENTS OF LABORATORY QUALITY SYSTEM

The test or calibration laboratories while formulating their Quality Manual should be aware the quality system elements specifically concerned to the laboratory. The elements for laboratory quality system are laid down in the respective ISO/IEC Guide 25:1990 or the national standard followed by an accreditation body. These quality system elements are as follows (respective clause of the ISO/IEC guide 25 is also given) :

- Organization and Management (Clause 4)
- Quality System Audit and Review (Clause 5)
- Records (Clause 12)
- Subcontracting of Calibration and Testing (Clause 14)

- Outside Support Services (Clause 15)
- Complaints (Clause 16)

The quality system elements form very important part of the Laboratory Quality Manual.

The each element of the applicable guide or standard may be addressed in separate chapter or section. The description of the element should be appropriate, while being logically and practically implementable in quality system. It may consist of the following:

Purpose of the Quality System Element

It should clearly state the necessity of the element in the Quality Manual.

Scope of Quality System Element

This means the applicability of the element.

Authority and Responsibility

The authority and responsibility to implement the related procedure associated with the element

Applicable Procedure

It should be clearly stated in different successive steps regarding "what is to be done and how is it to be done." The reference of corresponding specific quality system procedure applicable to met the requirement of the quality system element should be mentioned.

Documentation

The quality documents and records related to the quality system element, recording and storage and security of documents should be appropriately identified.

10.3.1 The Quality System Requirements for Laboratory Accreditation as Specified in the Latest Standard ISO 17025:1999 are as Follows

- Management Requirements
- Organization
- Quality System
- Document Control
- Review of Request, Tendering and Contracts
- Subcontracting of Test or Calibration
- Purchasing Services and Supplies
- Complaints
- Service to the Clients
- Control of nonconforming test and /or calibration work

- Corrective Action
- Preventive Action
- Control of Records
- Internal Audits
- Management Review

The latest standard ISO 17025:1999 for operation and technical competence of test or calibration laboratory has included the new clauses aligning this standard with ISO 9001 and ISO 9002 quality assurance standards. These clauses include quality system elements of laboratory accreditation which are explained as follows.

Document Control

The laboratory should address the requirements of the latest standard in the manual. The document control is essential to ensure that the correct procedure is being followed by the test or calibration personnel. The document control includes a well defined numbering system, approval, authorization and issue of reviewed, reaffirmed, amended documentation for implementation by the concerned.

Review of Request, Tendering and Contracts

The laboratory should address this element in its Quality Manual to acquaint the customer with the capability of the laboratory to perform the requisite tests as per the need of the client.

The terms and conditions of the contract should be described in the procedure. The client who floated a tender for testing of samples should also describe his implied and intended requirements before the final agreement for executing the contract.

The tendering or contract procedure should also describe the review mechanism for such contract.

Purchasing Services and Supplies

This element is of importance and the laboratory should address in Quality Manual its policy for procurement of new equipment, vendors whenever there is improvement in test method and higher accuracy equipment for such methods are available. The laboratory should describe its purchase procedure for vendor selection for laboratory consumables. The laboratory also describes its policy and procedure for availing the services of vendors for maintenance or calibration of instrumentation used in the laboratory.

Service to the Client

This element is a part of the commitment of the laboratory services to the client. The laboratory should address this element in the manual describing the procedure to consider the client's request for testing its sample in normal way, on priority or as per specified condition of procedure. If the clients require witnessing of any test, he should be welcome. The views of the clients for improvement in laboratory services should be well taken. The members of accreditation bodies or their representatives should be given proper attention on their visit and should be allowed to collect information if necessary.

Control of Non-Conforming Testing and/or Calibration Work

The laboratory should address its policy and procedure in the Quality Manual for controlling the nonconforming testing or calibration work related quality system and technical competence. The laboratory should describe in detail the quality system procedure developed for this element. To make it more clear it may be described in the quality system procedure that certain item or samples which are found nonconforming to the specified requirements are held for further processing and tested in accordance with the laboratory's in house test methods or customer's method or nonstandard methods on clearance from the authorized representative. The laboratory should maintain a separate record for such nonconforming testing or calibration work.

Corrective Action

This element is of utmost importance and the laboratory should describe in its Quality Manual the time bound procedure to take corrective action on a nonconformity observed during the internal audit or external audit of the laboratory.

Preventive Action

This element should be described in the manual highlighting the preventive action to avoid a recurring problem in testing or calibration items or in quality procedures/ standard operating procedures. The quality system procedure should be formulated by the concerned laboratory to find out the cause of recurring problem related to technical competence.

Thus the laboratory should align their Quality Manual to the elements of quality system as specified in the latest ISO 17025:1999 standard for laboratory accreditation.

10.4 ELEMENTS FOR TECHNICAL COMPETENCE OF LABORATORY

The technical competence elements as described in the ISO/IEC Guide 25:1990 are generally addressed in the Quality Manual by the concerned testing or calibration laboratory. The technical elements, before they are described in the Quality Manual by the laboratory, should have clarity for the following:

1. Purpose of technical element
2. Scope of technical element
3. Responsibility to implement the related technical element
4. Applicable procedure or SOP
5. Documentation

These technical competence elements are mentioned in chapter 2, but in brief are as follows:

- Personnel (clause 6)
- Accommodation and environment (clause 7)
- Measurement traceability and calibration (clause 9)
- Calibration and test methods (clause 10)
- Handling of test or calibration item (clause 11)
- Certificates and reports (clause 12)

10.4.1 The Technical Competence Requirements to be Addressed in the Quality Manual in Accordance with Latest ISO 17025:1999 Standard for Laboratory Accreditation

These are as follows:

- Technical requirements— General and specific factors affecting reliability of test or calibration
- Personnel
- Accommodation and environmental conditions
- Test and calibration method and method validation
- Equipment
- Measurement traceability
- Sampling
- Handling of test and calibration items
- Assuring the quality of test and calibration results
- Reporting the results

and special comments are due on the following.

Method Validation

Although this element was mentioned in ISO guide 25:1990 but the new standard ISO 17025:1999 has more emphasis on method validation. Therefore test or calibration laboratory should reflect this element in the Quality Manual of the laboratory and should develop a quality system procedure to validate the test methods in case it is developed by the laboratory itself or nonstandard methods are used by the laboratory on demand from the clients.

Sampling

The laboratory should address this element in the manual wherever the laboratory is involved in the sampling. The laboratory should have detailed sampling plans (single, double or multiple sampling plans) mentioning acceptance and rejection criteria.

Assuring the Quality of Test and Calibration Results

This element should be addressed in the manual stating the quality control, SQC, verification practices, repeat or replicate testing, inter/intra laboratory comparisons.

10.5 LISTING OF LABORATORY QUALITY SYSTEM PROCEDURES

The Quality Manual can be a compilation of all quality system procedures related to each element of quality system as well as technical competence. Thus listing of quality system procedures in the Quality Manual becomes essential. The quality system procedures should be given appropriate code and numbered. The cross-reference of quality procedures should be given in the manual by giving reference number to quality procedure applicable to a specific activity.

10.6 CROSS REFERENCING OF STANDARD OPERATING PROCEDURES

The documented Standard Operating Procedures are part of quality system for technical elements addressed in the Quality Manual for test or calibration methods. The Standard Operating Procedures should be clearly coded and numbered for identification. But the cross-referencing of individual Standard Operating Procedure in the manual is a difficult task for the laboratory as the number of Standard Operating Procedures followed by the laboratories for test or calibration methods is quite large.

Thus the test or calibration laboratory can give cross-reference of Standard Operating Procedure in specific cases if necessary. The listing of all Standard Operating Procedures in Quality Manual unnecessarily will be an attempt resulting in a very bulky manual. But the laboratory should have a control on these SOPs as they are the confidential technical information of the laboratories and can be made available to clients on special request.

10.7 EXAMPLES OF CONTENT LIST

Four examples of content list of Quality Manual of laboratories are presented in the boxes, as follows.

Example 10.1: Contents based on elements of ISO guide 25:1990
Example 10.2: Contents based on clause wise elements of ISO guide 25:1990
Example 10.3: Contents based on elements of standard ISO 17025:1999
Example 10.4: Contents based on clause wise elements of standard ISO 17025:1999

EXAMPLE 10.1

CONTENTS BASED ON ELEMENTS OF ISO GUIDE 25:1990

RTLL : Quality Manual	Page No:
Chapter : CONTENT	Revision No: Issue No : Date :

0.0	General
1	Organization and management
2	Quality system audit and review
3	Personnel
4	Accommodation and environment
5	Equipment and reference material
6	Measurement traceability and calibration
7	Calibration and test methods
8	Handling of test and calibration item
9	Certificates and reports
10	Records
11	Subcontracting of calibration and tests
12	Outside support services
13	Complaints

EXAMPLE 10.2

CONTENTS BASED ON CLAUSE WISE ELEMENTS OF ISO GUIDE 25:1990

RTLL : Quality Manual	Page No: Revision No: Issue No : Date :
Section: CONTENT	Page:

0.0	General
0.1	Amendment sheet
0.2	Distribution list
0.3	Abbreviation
0.4	Definition
1.0	Introduction
1.1	General Introduction
1.2	Purpose of Manual
1.3	Scope of this Manual
1.4	Administration of this manual
1.5	Field of activities
2.0	Quality Policy
2.1	Objective and commitment
3.0	Organization and management
3.1	Legal identity
3.2	Job description of technical manager
3.3	Job description of quality manager
3.4	Job description of chief chemist
3.5	Job description of chemist/analyst
3.6	Job description of quality executive
3.7	Job description of junior chemist/analyst
3.8	Independence of judgement
3.9	Confidentiality
3.10	Supervision accuracy
3.11	Improper influence
3.12	Confidentiality of clients proprietary rights and information
3.13	Nomination of deputies
3.14	Departure from documented policy and procedures
3.15	Organization chart

3.16	Commencement of new work
3.17	Document control
4.0	Quality system
4.1	Quality system documentation
4.2	Quality system audit
4.3	Corrective action
4.4	Reporting of audit and corrective action
4.5	Quality system review and reporting of review findings
5.0	Laboratory quality checks
5.1	Use of quality control practices
5.2	Retest or replicate testing
5.3	SQC Techniques
5.4	Alternate calculations
5.5	Inter-laboratory comparisons
6.0	Personnel
6.1	Qualification and experience
6.2	Training of personnel
6.3	Training records
7.0	Accommodation and environment
7.1	Laboratory accommodation
7.2	Laboratory environment and monitoring
7.3	Laboratory controlled areas
7.4	Good laboratory house keeping
8.0	Equipment and reference material
8.1	Use of equipment Outside permanent control
8.2	Equipment maintenance history and procedures
8.3	Equipment record
8.4	Reference material
8.5	Use of reference material Outside permanent control
8.6	Equipment calibration status and labeling
8.7	Reference material labeling and calibration status
8.8	Reference material records
9.0	Measurement traceability and calibration
9.1	Test equipment calibration /and verification programme
9.2	Calibration certificate
9.3	Uncertainty of measurement for test
9.4	Proficiency testing
9.5	Reference standards of measurement
9.6	Calibration programme for reference standards
9.7	In-service checks for calibration and verification
9.8	Reference standards traceability

10.0	Calibration and test methods
10.1	Work instruction for equipment preparation
10.2	Work instruction for sample preparation
10.3	Standard test methods for testing
10.4	Nonstandard method's validation and client agreement
10.6	Updating the test method and validation
10.7	Integrity of data and its transfer
10.8	Use of computers and security of data
10.9	Purchasing of consumables and storage
11.0	Handling of test and calibration item
11.1	Identification and recodification of test items
11.2	Procedures for environmental control during storage
11.3	Disposal of test item
12.0	Records
12.1	Record system and retention
12.2	Safety and security of records
13.0	Certificates and reports
13.1	Test reports/test results
13.2	Test certificate format detail
13.3	Incorporation of subcontracted test results
13.4	Duplicate test certificate provision
13.5	Control of dispatch of defective test results
13.6	Electronic transmission of test results
14.0	Subcontracting of testing
14.1	Subcontracted laboratory's compliance to standard
14.2	Record of subcontracted laboratories
15.0	Outside support services and supplies
15.1	Quality of vendors
15.2	Purchase procedures for equipment and materials
15.3	Suppliers' records
16.0	Complaint
16.1	Complaint redressel procedure
16.2	Audit against complaint
16.3	Complaints record

EXAMPLE 10.3

CONTENTS BASED ON ELEMENTS OF CONTENTS OF ISO 17025:1999 STANDARD

RTLL : Quality Manual	Page No:
Chapter : CONTENT	Revision No: Issue No : Date :

0.0	General
1	Management requirements
2	Organization
3	Quality system
4	Document control
5	Review of request, tendering and contracts
6	Subcontracting of tests and calibration
7	Purchasing services and supplies
8	Complaints
9	Service to the client
10	Control of nonconforming testing and/or calibration work
11	Corrective action
12	Preventive action
13	Control of records
14	Internal audits
15	Management review
16	Technical requirements
17	Personnel
18	Accommodation and environmental conditions
19	Test and calibration method and method validation
20	Equipment
21	Measurement traceability
22	Sampling
23	Handling of test and calibration item
24	Assuring the quality of test and calibration results
25	Reporting the results

EXAMPLE 10.4

CONTENTS BASED ON CLAUSE WISE ELEMENTS OF ISO STANDARD 17025:1999

RTLL : Quality Manual	Page No: Revision No: Issue No : Date :
Section: CONTENT	Page:

3.14	Supervision accuracy
3.15	Improper influence
3.16	Confidentiality of client's proprietary rights and information
3.17	Nomination of deputies
3.18	Departure from documented policy and procedures
4.0	Quality system
4.1	Quality system policies
4.2	Quality system objectives
4.3	Quality system documentation structure
4.4	Reference to quality system documents
5.0	Document control
5.1	Document approval and Issue
5.2	Document control procedures
5.3	Document change and control in computerized documentation
5.4	Document identification
6.0	Review of request of client for test
6.1	Client's tender for testing
6.2	Review of tender
6.3	Review of contract
6.4	Communication to client
6.5	Records of reviews
7.0	Subcontracting of testing
7.1	Selection of subcontracting laboratories
7.2	Subcontracted laboratory's compliance to the standard
7.3	Record of subcontracted laboratories
8.0	Purchasing services and supplies
8.1	Selection of purchase services and supplies
8.2	Compliance of supplied consumables to specification
8.3	Purchase order and review
8.4	Supplier's evaluation for critical consumables
8.5	Records of suppliers
9.0	Service to the client
9.1	Access of the client to the laboratory
9.2	Witnessing of test by the client
9.3	Communication to the client
9.4	Other feedback from the client
10.0	Complaint
10.1	Complaint redressel procedure
10.2	Investigation against complaint
10.3	Complaints record

11.0	Policy for control of nonconforming testing or calibration work
11.1	Management of nonconforming work
11.2	Evaluation of nonconforming work
11.3	Responsibility for resumption of nonconforming work
11.4	Corrective action for recurring nonconforming work
12.0	Corrective action policy
12.1	Authority to implement corrective action
12.2	Cause analysis
12.3	Selection and implementation of corrective action
12.4	Monitoring of corrective action
12.5	Additional audit for noncomplying activity
13.0	Preventive action
13.1	Identification of sources of preventive action
13.2	Preventive action plan
13.3	Preventive action record
14.0	Control of records
14.1	Indexing of records
14.2	Retention of records
14.3	Disposal of quality and technical records
14.4	Storage and security of records
14.5	Technical records
14.6	Identification of data for specific task
14.7	Data correction control in records
15.0	Internal audits
15.1	Internal audit plan
15.2	Internal auditor's qualification and training
15.3	Internal audit periodicity
15.4	Record of audit findings
15.5	Record of corrective action for audit findings
15.6	Follow up action on audit record
16.0	Management review
16.1	Management review committee
16.2	Review agenda
16.3	Periodicity of review
16.4	Records of review
16.5	Follow-up of review decisions
17.0	Technical requirements
17.1	General factors for correctness and reliability of test or calibration
17.2	Specific factors affecting test or calibration reliability
18.0	Personnel
18.1	Personnel qualification and experience

18.2	Identification of training needs
18.3	Competence and supervision of contracted personnel
18.4	Job description of personnel
18.5	Authorization of personnel for operation of specific equipment
18.6	Authorization of personnel to issue test reports
18.7	Records of training and authorization
19.0	Accommodation and environmental conditions
19.1	Laboratory accommodation
19.2	Laboratory environment
19.3	Environment control and monitoring
19.4	Records of environment control and monitoring
19.5	Control of cross contamination
19.6	Control of access to restricted areas
19.7	Good house keeping
20.0	Test or calibration method and method validation
20.1	Standard method
20.2	Selection of methods
20.3	Communication to client for use of selected method
20.4	Method developed by laboratory
20.5	Nonstandard method
20.6	Agreement with client for use of nonstandard method
20.7	Validation of methods
20.8	Method validation procedures
20.9	Records of validation of methods
21.0	Estimation of uncertainty of measurement
21.1	Internal calibration's uncertainty of measurement
21.2	Identification of component of uncertainty for specific cases
21.3	Methods of analysis of uncertainty
21.4	Records of uncertainty of measurement
22.0	Control of data
22.1	Checks on data transfer
22.2	Use of computer for data
22.3	Validation of computer software
22.4	Procedure for data protection and confidentiality
23.0	Equipment
23.1	Use of equipment outside permanent control
23.2	Accuracy compliance of equipment and software with test specification
23.3	Calibration programme for key items of equipment
23.4	Authorization of personnel for operation and maintenance of equipment
23.5	Identification of equipment and software items
23.6	Equipment's safe handling transport and storage

23.7	Equipment's maintenance planning
23.8	Identification and labeling of defective equipment
23.9	Equipment calibration status and labeling
23.10	Equipment's calibration checks before use
23.11	Intermediate calibration checks and records
23.12	Calibration copies correction
23.13	Equipment and software records
23.14	Equipment's safety from adjustment
23.15	Identification of equipment's software items
24.0	Measurement traceability
24.1	Equipment calibration programme
24.2	Traceability to SI units
24.3	Measurement uncertainty in calibration certificate
24.4	Compliance statement to metrological specification
24.5	Traceability to non SI units
24.6	Participation in inter-laboratory comparison
25.0	Testing
25.1	Test measurement traceability to SI units
25.2	Uncertainty of measurement for testing
25.3	Test measurement traceability to non SI units
26.0	Reference standard and reference material
26.1	Calibration programme for reference standards
26.2	Calibration traceability for reference standards
26.3	Calibration of reference standard on adjustment
26.4	Reference material traceability to SI units or CRM
26.5	Intermediate checks for reference standard or reference material or standard reference material
26.6	Transport and storage of reference standard or material
27.0	Sampling
27.1	Sampling plan and procedure
27.2	Deviation in sampling plan on consumers request
27.3	Sampling record
28.0	Handling of test and calibration items
28.1	Transportation procedure
28.2	Sample receipt procedure
28.3	Sample handling procedure
28.4	Sample protection and storage
28.5	Sample retention and disposal
28.6	Sample identification
28.7	Abnormality recording of test or calibration item on receipt
28.8	Sample handling instruction
28.9	Security and storage of secured items

29.0	Assuring the quality of test and calibration
29.1	Quality control for validity of test or calibration
29.2	Use of SQC techniques
29.3	Use of CRM (certified reference material) or SRM (standard reference material)
29.4	Replicate test by same or different method
29.5	Retest or re-calibration of items
29.6	Correlation of results for different characteristics of items
29.7	Proficiency testing
30.0	Reporting of results
30.1	Test or calibration reports for internal clients
30.2	Test report and calibration certificate requirement
30.3	Additional information on test report
30.4	Additional calibration certificate
30.5	Compliance to metrological specification
30.6	Report of calibration on adjustment
30.7	Calibration interval on certificate
30.8	Opinions and interpolations
30.9	Subcontractor's test or calibration results
30.10	Electronic transmission of test or calibration results
30.11	Test report or calibration certificate format
30.12	Amendment to test report or calibration certificate

11

Approval, Issue Amendment and Control of Quality Manual

11.1 APPROVING AUTHORITY FOR INITIAL QUALITY MANUAL AND THE REVISIONS

The laboratory quality manual which is developed with the participation of all concerned laboratory test or calibration personnel requires its approval from a person who is conversant with this activity and should be generally a senior person of the top management.

But this practice can only be followed by the laboratories which are of large size and possess larger hierarchy in the organizational structure.

Normally the top management of large sized laboratory approves the Quality Manual and authorizes the quality manager to approve the other quality documentation related to laboratory and also to coordinate the development of quality system documentation for the laboratory.

It is common experience that medium and small sized test or calibration laboratories face problems in approving the Quality Manual when the quality manager cum technical himself or herself develops the manual. In this situation, the test or calibration laboratory should clearly decide who should approve the manual. The problem can be solved if the manual is prepared by a third person working with the laboratory who is also familiar with the laboratory accreditation, and evaluated by the quality manager for its compliance to the accreditation elements as laid down in the latest accreditation criteria or standard. The third person can be authorized by the owner of the laboratory to prepare the quality manual and the quality –cum-technical manager can be authorized to approve the Quality Manual.

A laboratory quality manual on its revision can be approved by the top management or by quality manager in case authorized by the management.

11.2 ISSUING AUTHORITY FOR THE INITIAL AND REVISED QUALITY MANUAL

The issuance of the Quality Manual to the concerned does not only need a control of the manual but also requires the necessary procedure as to whom the manual be issued and who should issue. Generally the manual should be issued to all who are concerned for securing their contribution to quality of test or calibration of items. The manual issued to the associated laboratory personnel or external agencies should be controlled through a well controlled mechanism.

The quality manager in general is authorized by the top management to issue the manual to concerned laboratory personnel and external agencies, but in some cases it has been noticed that the chief executive issues it. In some cases the manuals have statements like "This manual issues with the approval of the chief executive or managing director".

11.3 AMENDMENT AND APPROVAL

The amendment to a laboratory quality manual can be initiated when it is observed that a particular clause or subclause related to a quality system element or technical element is not appropriately complying to the laid down requirements in the accreditation criteria or the national regulation or international standard.

The amendment to the Quality Manual can be made if it is practically established through systematic assessment that the description of a statement under some clause is ambiguous and not required under the respective quality system or technical element of accreditation.

The amendment in the manual can also be brought in if there are certain changes made in the national level regulations or international laboratory accreditation standard.

These amendments should be prepared by the concerned laboratory personnel responsible for quality system or technical elements of accreditation. After preparation, these amendments should be discussed with the concerned quality manager or technical manager along with the concerned supervisors. The amendment, if consensually accepted by the concerned, should be approved by the authorized quality manager and issued to the holder of the Quality Manual. The receipt of such amendments from the holder of the manual should be kept for document control function. The necessary changes should be made in the amendment sheet attached with the manual and latest amendment should be inserted by the concerned holder of the manual.

The Quality Manual should be revised in case the number of amendments exceeds a number between 10 to 15, as determined by the laboratory. Efforts should be made by the laboratory to implement effectively the revised Quality Manual.

11.4 CONTROL OF LABORATORY QUALITY MANUAL

The Quality Manual, which is key document for establishing and maintaining the quality system of laboratory, should not only be controlled but also have appropriate distribution system.

The Quality Manual's all pages covering different sections related to various quality system element or technical requirements should have a unique page numbering system so that a page from a particular section can be replaced and subsequently inserted on some amendment. This can be achieved through a document control procedure maintained in the laboratory for incorporation of such amendments made from time to timc. For clarity regarding changes in the manual a method to highlight the actual changes should be used.

To maintain up-to-date current position of the laboratory quality manual, a method to assure change receipt and insertion in the manual by the manual holder should be used by the laboratory. For example the revised pages for some amendment may be accompanied by some attributory note receipt system under which the receipt is signed by the recipient as certificate of change or amendment's receipt and incorporation. These receipts are then collected for document control functions. An appropriate amendment to the table of contents may be added to assure the user of the latest revision of the Quality Manual.

Before finalization, publication and issuance of the Quality Manual, the document should be presented to the representative of the laboratory's senior management for final review, suitability and appropriate structure. The intended internal or external user of manual should also have an opportunity to comment on the usability.

The internal distribution of the manual should be such that every user has the access to the manual. All the copies issued to the concerned should have serial numbers with a provision of record of receipt of the same. The laboratory management should ensure that every internal user of the manual is fully acquainted with the content and the use of the laboratory quality manual.

The copies of Quality Manual distributed to internal user or sent to an accreditation body for grant of accreditation should be marked as "CONTROLLED COPY" and for other external users it should be marked as "UNCONTROLLED COPY".

12

How to Write Laboratory Quality Manual

12.1 INTRODUCTION

As and when the top management of the test or calibration laboratory has decided to adopt laboratory quality system based on ISO/IEC Guide 25:1990 or international standard ISO 17025:1999, it is the utmost duty of the top management of the laboratory to nominate or appoint a laboratory quality manager to write and coordinate the quality related activities in the laboratory.

While writing the quality manual, almost all quality managers face the synonymous common problem. Most of the laboratories attempt to get the quick results and appoint consultants for writing the Quality Manual. The manual written by these consultants are normally generic, formal or sometimes become too perfect which is tantamount to a document aimed to achieve accreditation by any way.

The laboratory quality manual is a most practical document and it should clearly address the laboratory quality policy, quality procedures and standard operating procedures. The quality procedures and Standard Operating Procedures should be clear, most accurate, concise and understandable to the user.

The test or calibration laboratories are mostly involved in serving the internal or external clients. This aspect of client service or commercial services should also be reflected in the documented form in the Quality Manual.

Therefore the writing of Quality Manual by the consultants should be avoided by the laboratories and involve all concerned personnel in the manual preparation. Based upon the experience and guide lines the following sixteen step procedure for writing Quality Manual is recommended. These are only the guide lines to facilitate the quality managers or writers of the manual. Every test or calibration laboratory or writer of the Quality Manual may adopt his or her style to meet the specific requirements of laboratory accreditation. Overview of major stages in development of laboratory quality manual is at Fig. 12.1.

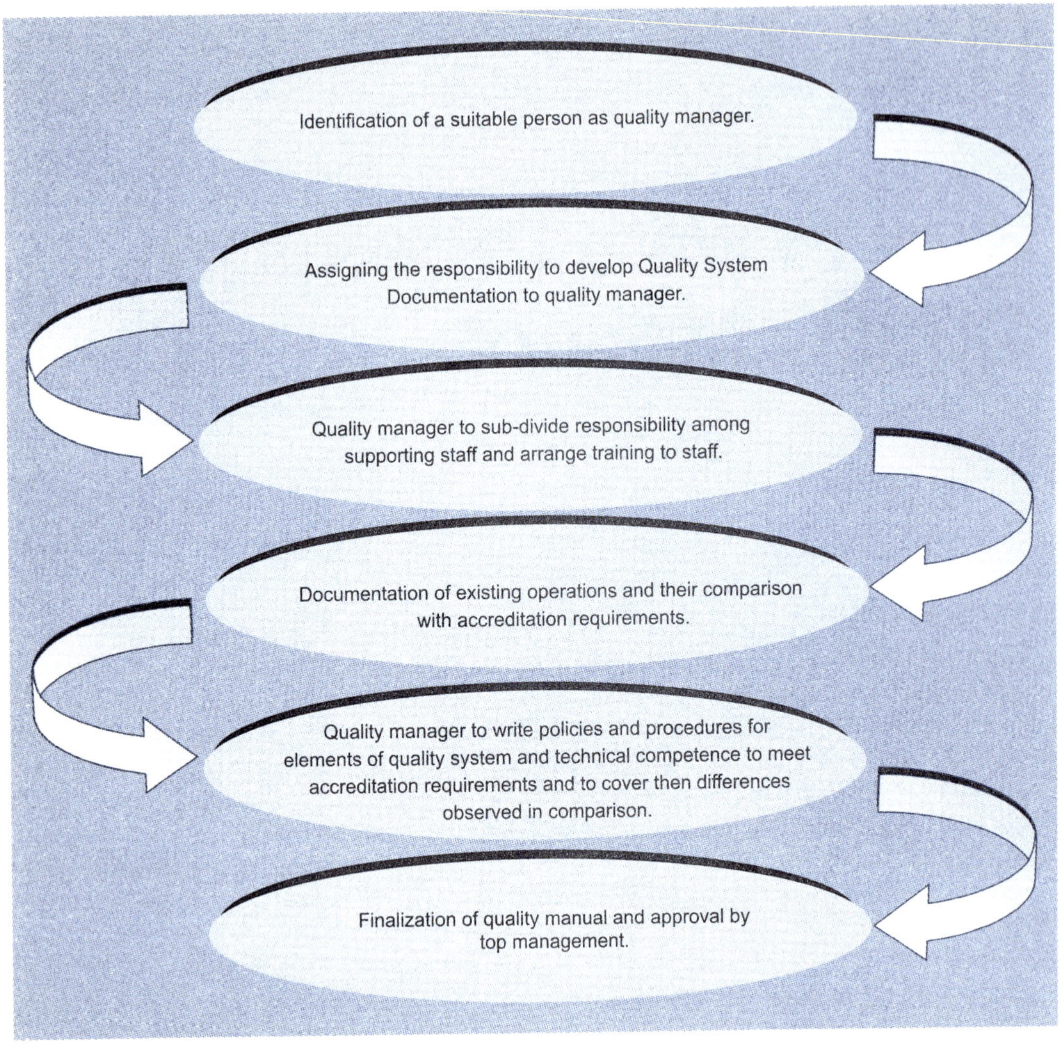

Fig. 12.1: *Major stages in development of laboratory quality manual*

12.2 STEPS IN WRITING QUALITY MANUAL

Step 1 Determine which specific criteria for test or calibration along with ISO/IEC Guide 25:1990 or latest standard ISO 17025:1999 (General Requirements for Competence of Testing or Calibration Laboratories) are suitable to your laboratory.

Step 2 Draft the section wise content of Quality Manual complying to the requirements of ISO/IEC Guide 25:1990 or ISO 17025:1999 and the specific criteria.

Step 3 Identify and list the quality system procedure related to each section of the manual.

Step 4 Identify and list standard operating procedures related to specific section of the manual.

Step 5 Classify the organization of the laboratory in to functional groups for quality system and technical competence related activities.

Step 6 Allocate the quality manual, quality procedures and standard operating Procedures writing task to these functional groups.

Step 7 Determine the structure of the quality manual. Design format of manual, quality procedures and standard operating procedures. Adopt some suitable numbering system for quality procedures and standard operating procedures.

Step 8 Train the test or calibration personnel engaged in document formulation on how to write and how to organize.

The familiarity of the personnel with ISO/IEC Guide 25:1990 or ISO 17025:1999 and ISO guide 49:1986 (Guide to write Quality Manual) shall be helpful.

Step 9 List out existing quality procedures and standard operating procedures in practice and review them to align with the requisite format of quality procedures and standard operating procedures.

Step 10 Prepare check list and appropriate questionnaire to collect essential information for writing quality manual, quality procedures and standard operating procedures.

Step 11 Collect and compile the information through discussion and interviews.

Step 12 Write down draft quality manual in the designed standard format based upon the collected information.

Step 13 Compile the quality manual, quality procedures and standard operating procedures in standardized form.

Step 14 Organize a review of the draft Quality Manual with test or calibration personnel to whom the writing task had been assigned and the would be user. Identify essential corrections to be made.

Step 15 Incorporate the corrections and prepare a final copy of the Quality Manual.

Step 16 Take approval of top management and authorization (for printing and distribution of manual to the concerned as per the manual control procedure.

13

Action Plan to Write Laboratory Quality Manual

The test or calibration laboratory should follow the action plan for writing the Quality Manual.

13.1 Step 1

Determine which specific criteria for test or calibration along with ISO/IEC Guide 25:1990 or ISO 17025:1999 standard (General requirements for competence of testing or calibration laboratories) are suitable to your laboratory.

The test or calibration laboratory should identify the specific criteria developed by the national accreditation body either for test or calibration. The specific criteria developed by the national accreditation body may be obtained for different areas of test or calibration, like -

1. *Testing:* chemical, microbiological, electronics, Mechanical, nondestructive testing, electrical or optical.
2. *Calibration:* mechanical measurement, thermal measurement, electrical measurement or optical measurement.

13.2 Step 2

Draft section-wise content of Quality Manual complying to the requirements of ISO/IEC Guide 25: 1990 or ISO 17025: 1999 standard and specific criteria.

After selecting the appropriate specific criteria for testing or calibration, it is desirable for the laboratory that the Quality Manual must address the generic requirement of quality system, technical competence and specific requirement of the relevant specific criteria.

A very simple method of sectionizing the content of the manual is that each accreditation element should be addressed in a single chapter. But it is not necessary that order of sections of manual is the same as that of the international standard.

For example

<table>
<tr><td colspan="2">RTLL :Quality Manual</td><td rowspan="2">Page No:
Revision No:
Issue No :
Date :</td></tr>
<tr><td colspan="2">Chapter : CONTENT</td></tr>
<tr><td>0.0</td><td colspan="2">General</td></tr>
<tr><td>1</td><td colspan="2">Management requirements</td></tr>
<tr><td>2</td><td colspan="2">Organization</td></tr>
<tr><td>3</td><td colspan="2">Quality system</td></tr>
<tr><td>4</td><td colspan="2">Document control</td></tr>
<tr><td>5</td><td colspan="2">Review of request, tendering and contracts</td></tr>
<tr><td>6</td><td colspan="2">Subcontracting of tests and calibration</td></tr>
<tr><td>7</td><td colspan="2">Purchasing services and supplies</td></tr>
<tr><td>8</td><td colspan="2">Complaints</td></tr>
<tr><td>9</td><td colspan="2">Service to the client</td></tr>
<tr><td>10</td><td colspan="2">Control of nonconforming testing and/or calibration work</td></tr>
<tr><td>11</td><td colspan="2">Corrective action</td></tr>
<tr><td>12</td><td colspan="2">Preventive action</td></tr>
<tr><td>13</td><td colspan="2">Control of records</td></tr>
<tr><td>14</td><td colspan="2">Internal audits</td></tr>
<tr><td>15</td><td colspan="2">Management review</td></tr>
<tr><td>16</td><td colspan="2">Technical requirements</td></tr>
<tr><td>17</td><td colspan="2">Personnel</td></tr>
<tr><td>18</td><td colspan="2">Accommodation and environmental conditions</td></tr>
<tr><td>19</td><td colspan="2">Test and calibration method and method validation</td></tr>
<tr><td>20</td><td colspan="2">Equipment</td></tr>
<tr><td>21</td><td colspan="2">Measurement traceability</td></tr>
<tr><td>22</td><td colspan="2">Sampling</td></tr>
<tr><td>23</td><td colspan="2">Handling of test and calibration item</td></tr>
<tr><td>24</td><td colspan="2">Assuring the quality of test and calibration results</td></tr>
<tr><td>25</td><td colspan="2">Reporting the results</td></tr>
</table>

13.3 Step 3

Identify and list the quality system procedures related to each section of the manual.

Quality system procedures are the important basis of the Quality Manual and are basic documentation used for the planning and implementation of quality system. Without appropriate numbering of quality procedures a Quality Manual can not be formulated. Therefore it is very much essential for the manual writer to identify and list out quality procedures to serve the purpose of the laboratory for implementation of quality system.

13.4 Step 4

Identify and list Standard Operating Procedures related to specific sections of the manual.

Standard Operating Procedures are very much essential for maintaining the technical competence of the test or calibration laboratory. There are numerous Standard Operating Procedures but the most important are concerned with test or calibration methods. Thus the manual writer should identify the needs for Standard Operating Procedures and list them in order as cross reference in the Quality Manual. The listing of all Standard Operating Procedures in the manual is not possible as it will only make the manual bulky.

13.5 Step 5

Classify the organization of laboratory into functional groups for quality system and technical competence related activities.

The test or calibration may be independent, commercial entity or it may be part of the industry. But every laboratory has its own organizational structure. The organization may possess different departments for test or calibration in various areas or it may have small section to carry out the task. Thus for the purpose of writing of the manual the test or calibration laboratory can be divided into the following functional groups:

- Quality system management
- Technical management
- Sample collection and receipt
- Equipment maintenance and calibration
- Purchase and subcontracting
- Stocking of consumables or samples
- Quality assurance

13.6 Step 6

Allocate the quality manual, quality procedures, and standard operating procedures writing tasks to these functional groups.

The responsibility for writing quality manual, quality procedures, standard operating procedures, quality records or work instructions should be assigned to the personnel directly associated with the functional groups. These test or calibration personnel should be given responsibility to write different chapters of the quality manual and their associated quality procedures or standard operating procedures. The quality manager should be responsible to coordinate these activities.

The assigned responsibilities to various personnel of functional groups is illustrated in Table 13.1.

13.7 Step 7

Determine the structure of the Quality Manual. Design a format of the manual, quality procedures and standard operating procedures. Adopt some suitable numbering system for quality procedures and standard operating procedures.

Structure of Quality Manual

There is no ISO standard available which defines the structure of laboratory's Quality Manual but such a manual should have the following :

General Information

The manual should have the general information of

- Manual's table of contents
- Scope of Quality Manual
- Introductory pages for laboratory and the company
- Manual issue number, date of issue
- Amendment status with record
- Authority to issue Quality Manual and respective amendments
- Glossary of standard terms used in the Quality Manual
- Distribution list

Elements of Laboratory Quality System

The manual should address each element of quality system in separate chapters. These chapters may have sub-content to meet the requirement of quality system element. The following information must be there :

- Quality system element description
- Scope of element
- Responsibility to document and maintain
- Description of systematic procedure to meet the requirement
- Reference of applicable quality system procedure
- Necessary documentation
- Records

Table 13.1: *Responsibility allocations of functional groups*

Functional Groups	*ISO 17025:1999 Requirements (clause wise)*	*Chapter No.*	*Personnel*
Quality System Management	Management requirements (Cl. 4)	1	
	Organization (Cl. 4.1)	2	
	Quality system (Cl. 4.2)	3	
	Document control (Cl. 4.3)	4	
	Internal audits (Cl. 4.13)	14	
	Management review (Cl. 4.14)	15	
Purchase and Sub-contracting	Review of request, tendering and contracts (Cl. 4.4)	5	
	Subcontracting of tests and calibration (Cl. 4.5)	6	
	Purchasing services and supplies (Cl. 4.6)	7	
Sample Collection and Receipt	Complaints (Cl. 4.8)	8	
	Service to clients (Cl. 4.7)	9	
	Control of nonconforming testing and/or calibration work (Cl. 4.9)	10	
	Corrective action (Cl. 4.10)	11	
	Preventive action (Cl. 4.11)	12	
	Control of records (Cl. 4.12)	13	
Technical Management	Technical requirements (Cl. 5 and 5.1)	16	
	Personnel (Cl. 5.2)	17	
	Accommodation and environmental conditions (Cl. 5.3)	18	
	Test or calibration method and method validation (Cl. 5.4)	19	
	Sampling (Cl. 5.7)	22	
Equipment Maintenance and Calibration	Equipment (Cl. 5.5) Measurement traceability (Cl. 5.6)	20 21	
Stocking of Consumables or Sample	Handling of test and calibration items	23	
Quality Assurance	Assuring the quality of test and calibration results (Cl. 5.9)	24	
	Reporting of results (Cl. 5.10)	25	

Elements of Technical Competence

The Quality Manual which is to be made on the basis of ISO/IEC Guide 25:1990 or ISO 17025:1999 should address all technical elements in separate chapters and related sub-content list may be used to meet the requirement of technical element.

- Technical element description
- Scope of element
- Responsibility to document and maintain
- Description of systematic procedure to meet the requirements
- Reference of applicable standard operating procedures
- Necessary documentation
- Records

Document Numbering System

The laboratory should adopt a unique numbering system to identify the various quality system documents. The document either may be identified by the suffix of the title of document or by a numerical number. The suitable numbering should be designed to suit the existing documentation system of the laboratory.

The quality system procedures or standard operating procedures numbering system should be such that it can be easily identified with the related section of the manual and have provision of further extension.

The laboratory should maintain a master register for appropriate record of quality system procedure and standard operating procedures.

Format of Quality Manual

The laboratory Quality Manual in general is written in a particular format and this format is followed for writing the matter dealing with a particular accreditation element. The each page of the manual consists of TOP CONTROL BOX at the top and BOTTOM CONTROL BOX at the bottom of the page.
The top control box should have the following information,

- Laboratory's name or Company's name
- Document's Name (Quality Manual)
- Title of Chapter
- Section No.
- Issue No.
- Revision No.
- Page No.

as follows-

Laboratory's Name	Quality Manual	Section No.: Issue No.: Revision No.: Date :
Chapter	Title of Element	Page 1 of 2

The bottom control box has the following information,

- Prepared by
- Approved by

as follows :

Prepared by: Approved by:

The above mentioned TOP and BOTTOM Control Boxes may be used by the laboratory for each page of the manual.

Annexure Section

The manual should have annexures for the following,

- List of quality system procedures
- Other associated information if necessary

13.8 Step 8

Train the test or calibration personnel in document formulation on how to write, what to write and how to organize.

As in preparation of quality system documentation for the laboratory, personnel from various sections or departments are involved, therefore it becomes necessary to train these personnel in document writing. As document writing is an art which may not be possible to acquire with out imparting training to technical personnel who have devoted lengthy time either in testing, calibration or field jobs.

ISO Guide 49:1986 provides certain guide lines to develop a Quality Manual for the laboratories. A review of this ISO guide may be helpful to associated test or calibration personnel for understanding how to write the quality documentation and Quality Manual.

The familiarity of personnel with ISO/IEC Guide 25:1990 or ISO 17025:1999 and ISO 49:1986 to write Quality Manual will be helpful. The responsibilities for laboratory quality system documentation and associated activities are mentioned in table no. 13.2.

13.9 Step 9

List out existing quality system procedures and standard operating procedures in practice and review them to align the requisite format of quality system procedure and standard operating procedures.

Table 13.2: *Responsibilities for laboratory quality system documentation and associated activites*

Levels of Laboratory Quality System Documentation	*Responsibility to write/organize*	*Activities*
Quality Manual (I)	Quality Manual	• Coordination • Organizing • Interviewing • Reviewing • Incorporating • Corrections • Documenting • Distribution
Quality Procedures (II)	Department, section heads, chief analyst or supervisor	• Identification • Purpose of quality procedures • Responsibility • Documenting • Discussions
Standard Operating Procedures (III)	Technical Manager or Chief Analyst	• Identification of SOPs • Purpose • Scope • Responsibility • SOPs writing • Discussion • Review
Quality Documents (IV)	Quality Assurance Manager, Supervisor	• Design of records, format, forms, report certificates, review reports • Other records

It is generally observed that any laboratory associated with a parent organization or functioning independently must be having certain quality system procedures or standard operating procedures in practice for day to day task. Therefore, these quality system procedures or standard operating procedures should be collected and reviewed to determine whether these QSOPs or SOPs are sufficient for present state of quality or they need some modification. Based on these reviews of quality system procedures and SOPs, an action plan can be prepared to collect and compile the quality system documentation.

13.10 Step 10

Prepare check lists and appropriate questionnaires to collect essential information for writing Quality Manual, Quality Procedures, Standard Operating Procedures.

For writing the Quality Manual, Quality Procedures, Standard Operating Procedures, a systematic stepwise technique should be adopted by the writers of these documents. The questionnaires or the check list based on the following questions for interviewing the concerned, should be prepared by the writers to collect the appropriate information :

- What is the purpose of a particular accreditation requirement?
- What action is required to meet the requirement?
- Why an action be taken?
- Where are the accreditation requirements met?
- When are the accreditation requirements met?
- Who is responsible for action completion?
- How is it done?
- Who are the internal or external customers?

These primary questions will help in reviewing the working practice of the laboratory and at the same time one can collect lot of information for writing the Quality Manual.

The examination of the questions will clearly show that the first question is related to an accreditation element and particularly to its PURPOSE.

The second question is related to the SCOPE of the accreditation element.

The thirds question relates to the response "that always has been done that way".

The fourth question relates to it better method by developing to "how else it can be completed".

The question related to "Who is responsible" should be replied by the designations of the personnel and not by their names to overcome the difficulty arising that whenever there would be a change in the personnel, a change in the manual is needed. An organization chart should be developed to explain the authority and responsibility of the personnel.

The reply to the question "how is it done" should be given by appropriate cross reference to quality system procedure in the manual or standard operating procedures reference.

A good Quality Manual should have cross reference of quality system procedures and standard operating procedures (specific only) and listing of quality system procedures to demonstrate the capability of laboratory with out disclosing the confidentiality and trade secrets to the clients or competitors.

13.11 Step 11

Collect and compile the information through discussion and interviews.

After preparing the check list related to quality system documentation, questionnaires should be circulated to the test or calibration personnel to provide the sufficient and appropriate information to the concerned writers of the Quality Manual, Quality System Procedures, or Standard Operating Procedures. The further detailed information may be collected through interviews, discussions directly with key personnel who are involved in quality related activities of the test or calibration laboratory and may be the user of Quality System Procedures, Standard Operating Procedures, and Quality Manual in future.

Thus the information so collected should be compiled to commence the writing of laboratory Quality System Documentation and Quality Manual in particular.

13.12 Step 12

Write down draft Quality Manual in the standard designed format based upon the collected information.

On collecting the requisite information, the test or calibration personnel who have already been assigned the responsibility to write Quality Manual, Quality Procedures, and Standard Operating Procedures, should start the writing of Quality Manual.

A typical Quality Manual complying to the clause-wise requirements of latest standard ISO 17025:1999 for laboratory accreditation can be formulated in 30 chapters (Example 13.1).

13.13 Step 13

Compile the Quality Manual, Quality Procedures, and Standard Operating Procedures in standardized form.

Since the writing of different chapters of the Quality Manual is done by the different personnel it is required to organize these chapters according to the content list. Each page of the Quality Manual should be either typed or hand written into a prescribed format for Quality Manual with appropriate document control at top and bottom.

While the writing of Quality Manual is done by various test or calibration personnel according to their assigned responsibility, the compilation of the manual in the standard form should be done by the appointed Quality Manager. All pages may be numbered in a loose leaf file system to provide quick removal of pages on amendment.

13.14 Step 14

Organize the review of draft Quality Manual with, the test or calibration personnel to whom the writing task is assigned, and the would-be users. Identify essential corrections to be made.

The draft laboratory Quality Manual as prepared should be reviewed to evaluate its compliance to the requirements of ISO 17025:1999 standard for laboratory accreditation.

The review meeting should comprise of all test or calibration personnel, future users and affected section of the laboratory.

The decision of the review meeting should be recorded and appropriate communication to all concerned should be made for necessary action at their end.

Example 13.1

COMPILATION OF CLAUSE REQUIREMENTS OF ISO 17025: 1999 STANDARD IN THE QUALITY MANUAL

CHAPTER	CLAUSE OF ISO 17025:1999
0.0	General
0.1	Amendment sheet
0.2	Distribution list
0.3	Abbreviation
0.4	Definition
1.0	Introduction
1.1	Purpose of manual
1.2	Scope of this manual
1.3	Administration of this manual
1.4	Field of activities
	4.2 Quality System
	(Clause 4.2.2)
2.0	Laboratory quality policy
2.1	Quality policy objective
2.2	Commitment to good professional practices
2.3	Commitment to laboratory's standard of services
2.4	Commitment to compliance to this standard
2.5	Familiarity with quality system documentation
	Clause 4: Management Requirements
3.0	Management requirements
	Clause 4.1 Organization
3.1	Organization and Management Structure
3.2	Laboratory's legal responsibility
3.3	Laboratory's status (Permanent, temporary, or mobile)
3.4	Conflict of interest
3.5	Technical management
3.6	Job description of Technical manager
3.7	Job description of quality manager
3.8	Independence of judgement
3.9	Confidentiality and integrity
3.10	Supervision adequacy
3.11	Improper influence
3.12	Confidentiality of clients

3.13	Proprietary rights and information
3.14	Nomination of deputies
3.15	Departure from documented policy and procedures
	Clause 4.2: Quality System
4.0	Quality system
4.1	Quality system policies
4.2	Quality system objectives
4.3	Quality system documentation structure
4.4	Reference to quality system documents
4.5	Quality system documentation communication and availability
	Clause 4.3: Document Control
5.0	Document control
5.1	Document approval and Issue
5.2	Document control procedures
5.3	Document change, review and reaffirmation
5.4	Document change and control in computerized documentation
5.5	Document identification
	Clause 4.4: Review of request, tender and contract
6.0	Review of request of client for test
6.1	Client's tender for testing
6.2	Review of tender
6.3	Review of contract
6.4	Communication to client
6.5	Records of reviews
	Clause 4.5: Subcontracting of test and calibration
7.0	Subcontracting testing
7.1	Selection of subcontracting laboratories
7.2	Subcontracted laboratory's Compliance to the standard
7.3	Record of subcontracted laboratories
	Clause 4.6 Purchasing services and supplies
8.0	Purchasing services and supplics
8.1	Selection of purchase services and supplies
8.2	Compliance of supplied consumables to specification
8.3	Purchase order and review
8.4	Supplier's evaluation for critical consumables
8.5	Records of suppliers
	Clause 4.7 Service to client
9.0	Service to the client
9.1	Access of the client to the laboratory
9.2	Witnessing of test by the client

9.3	Communication to the client
9.4	Other feedback from the client
	Clause 4.8 Complaints
10.0	Complaint
10.1	Complaint redressel procedure
10.2	Investigation against complaint
10.3	Complaints record
	Clause 4.9 Controlling of nonconforming testing and/or calibration work
11.0	Policy for control of nonconforming testing or calibration work
11.1	Management of nonconforming work
11.2	Evaluation of nonconforming work
11.3	Responsibility for resumption of nonconforming work
11.4	Corrective action for recurring nonconforming work
	Clause 4.10: Corrective action
12.0	Corrective action policy
12.1	Authority to implement corrective action
12.2	Cause analysis
12.3	Selection and implementation of corrective action
12.4	Monitoring of corrective action
12.5	Additional audit for noncomplying activity
	Clause 4.11 Preventive action
13.0	Preventive action
13.1	Identification of sources of preventive action
13.2	Preventive action plan
13.3	Preventive action procedure
13.4	Preventive action record
	Clause 4.12: Control of records
14.0	Control of records
14.1	Indexing of records
14.2	Retention of records
14.3	Disposal of quality and technical records
14.4	Storage and security of records
14.5	Technical records
14.6	Identification of data for specific task
14.7	Data correction control in records
	Clause 4.13: Internal Audits
15.0	Internal audits
15.1	Internal audit plan
15.2	Internal auditor's qualification and training

15.3	Internal audit periodicity
15.4	Record of audit findings
15.5	Record of corrective action for audit findings
15.6	Follow up action on audit record
	Clause 4.14 Management Review
16.0	Management review
16.1	Management review committee
16.2	Review agenda
16.3	Periodicity of review
16.4	Records of review
16.5	Follow-up of review decision
	Clause 5: Technical Requirements
17.0	Technical requirements
	Clause 5.1 General
17.1	General factors for correctness and reliability of test or calibration
17.2	Specific factors affecting test or calibration reliability
	Clause 5.2 : Personnel
18.0	Personnel
18.1	Personnel qualification and experience
18.2	Identification of training needs
18.3	Competence and supervision of contracted personnel
18.4	Job description of personnel
18.5	Authorization of personnel for operation of specific equipment
18.6	Authorization of personnel to issue test reports
18.7	Records of training and authorization
	Clause 5.3: Accommodation and Environment
19.0	Accommodation and environmental conditions
19.1	Laboratory accommodation
19.2	Laboratory environment
19.3	Environment control and monitoring
19.4	Records of environment control and monitoring
19.5	Control of cross contamination
19.6	Control of access to restricted areas
19.7	Good house keeping
	Clause 5.4 : Test and calibration methods and method validation
20.0	Test or calibration method and method validation
20.1	Standard method
20.2	Selection of methods
20.3	Communication to client for use of selected method
20.4	Method developed by laboratory

20.5	Nonstandard method
20.6	Agreement with client for use of nonstandard method
20.7	Validation of methods
20.8	Method validation procedures
20.9	Records of validation of methods
	Clause 4.5.6 : Estimation of uncertainty of measurement
21.0	Estimation of uncertainty of measurement
21.1	Internal calibration's uncertainty of measurement
21.2	Identification of component of uncertainty for specific cases
21.3	Methods of analysis of uncertainty
21.4	Records of uncertainty of measurement
	Clause 4.5.7: Control of data
22.0	Control of data
22.1	Checks on data transfer
22.2	Use of computer for data
22.3	Validation of computer software
22.4	Procedure for data protection and confidentiality
	Clause 5.5 : Equipment
23.0	Equipment
23.1	Use of equipment Outside permanent control
23.2	Accuracy compliance of equipment and software with test specification
23.3	Calibration programme for key items of equipment
23.4	Authorization of personnel for operation and maintenance of equipment
23.5	Identification of equipment and software items
23.6	Equipment's safe handling transport and storage
23.7	Equipment's maintenance planning
23.8	Identification and labeling of defective equipment
23.9	Equipment calibration status and labeling
23.10	Equipment's calibration checks before use
23.11	Intermediate calibration checks and records
23.12	Calibration copies correction
23.13	Equipment and software records
23.14	Equipment's safety from adjustment
23.15	Identification of equipment's software items
	Clause 5.6: Measurement Traceability
	Clause 5.6.1 General
24.0	Measurement traceability
	Clause 5.6.2 Specific Requirement (Calibration)
24.1	Equipment calibration programme

24.2	Traceability to SI units
24.3	Measurement uncertainty in calibration certificate
24.4	Compliance statement to metrological specification
24.5	Traceability to non SI units
24.6	Participation in inter-laboratory comparisons
	Clause 5.6.2.2: Testing
25.0	Testing
25.1	Test measurement traceability to SI units
25.2	Uncertainty of measurement for test
25.3	Test measurement traceability to non SI units
	Clause 5.6.3: Reference standards and reference materials
26.0	Reference standard and reference material
26.1	Calibration programme for reference standards
26.2	Calibration traceability for reference standards
26.3	Calibration of reference standard on adjustment
26.4	Reference material traceability to SI units or CRM
26.5	Intermediate checks for reference standard or reference material or SRM
26.6	Transport and storage of reference standard or material
	Clause 5.7: Sampling
27.0	Sampling
27.1	Sampling plan and procedure
27.2	Deviation in sampling plan on consumers request
27.3	Sampling record
	Clause 5.8: Handling of test and calibration items
28.0	Handling of test and calibration items
28.1	Transportation procedure
28.2	Sample receipt procedure
28.3	Sample handling procedure
28.4	Sample protection and storage
28.5	Sample retention and disposal
28.6	Sample identification
28.7	Abnormality recording of test or calibration item on receipt
28.8	Sample handling instruction
28.9	Security and storage of secured items
	Clause 5.9: Assuring the quality of test and calibration results
29.0	Assuring the quality of test and calibration
29.1	Quality control for validity of test or calibration
29.2	Use of SQC techniques
29.3	Use of CRM or SRM
29.4	Replicate test by same or different method

29.5	Retest or re-calibration of item
29.6	Correlation of results for different characteristics of items
29.7	Proficiency Testing
	Clause 5.10: Reporting the results
30.0	Reporting of results
30.1	Test or calibration reports for internal clients
30.2	Test report and calibration certificate requirement
30.3	Additional information on test report
30.4	Additional calibration certificate
30.5	Compliance to metrological specification
30.6	Report of calibration on adjustment
30.7	Calibration interval on certificate
30.8	Opinions and interpolations
30.9	Subcontractor's test or calibration results
30.10	Electronic transmission of test or calibration results
30.11	Test report or calibration certificate format
30.12	Amendment to test report or calibration certificate

13.15 Step 15

Incorporate the corrections and prepare a final copy of the Quality Manual.

The comments of the test or calibration and future users on adequacy of the Quality Manual to requirements of ISO 17025:1999 should be incorporated in the respective chapters. The verification of incorporation of such comments in the Quality Manual should be done by the quality manager.

The finalized Quality Manual is now ready for the approval or authorization by the top management.

13.16 Step 16

Take approval of top management and authorization for printing and distribution of manual to the concerned as per the manual control procedure.

The quality manager should take approval of the manual for printing, issuance and distribution to the concerned personnel. The control of the manual should be in accordance with the document control procedures of the laboratory.

14

A Guiding Sample For Laboratory Quality Manual

INTRODUCTION

This guiding sample for laboratory Quality Manual is formulated on the basis of study of large number of Quality Manuals related to test or calibration laboratories.

For writing the Quality Manual, there should be a cover page providing the name of the laboratory, name of the organization to which it belongs, title of the manual, approving and issuing authority, copy number, copy holder and issue number (Example 14.1).

Next, an authorization for release of Quality Manual should be inserted. It should carry the description of authority, e.g. head of organization, authorizing the release of the document (Example 14.2). The same should also be reflected on each page of the manual.

The manual should have the TOP (Document) CONTROL BOX and BOTTOM CONTROL BOX on each page. In this sample the bottom control box has not been shown on each page of the manual which needs to be taken care of by the concerned laboratories. This manual should not be taken up verbatim or copied by the laboratories. The laboratories may take help from it for developing their own Quality Manual and aligning the same with the requirements of latest standard ISO 17025:1999 of laboratory accreditation.

The contents of the manual (Example 14.3) are from the ISO 17025:1999. Attempts have been made to cover each and every clause of the latest standard for competence of the testing and calibration laboratories. The contents of the Quality Manual may be taken in the same order as given in the standard. But there is no hard and fast rule to follow the same order. It is left to the choice of the laboratory concerned.

Example 14.3 is then continued further with sectionwise elucidation, thus covering all the sections related to contents of the manual.

Example 14.1: *Sample Format for Quality Manual's Cover Page*

RAJSHREE TESTING LABORATORIES LTD.

QUALITY MANUAL
CONTROLLED COPY

Approved by:
Issued by:
Copy no.
Holder no.
Date   Issue no.

Example 14.2: *Sample Format of Quality Manual's Release Authorization Sheet*

RAJSHREE TESTING LABORATORIES LTD.

QUALITY MANUAL RELEASE AUTHORIZATION

THIS QUALITY MANUAL HAS BEEN RELEASED UNDER THE AUTHORITY OF (NAME AND DESIGNATION OF HEAD OF ORGANIZATION).

IT IS PROPERTY OF (LABORATORY' NAME WITH ADDRESS)

SIGNATURE
NAME :
DESIGNATION:

Approved by:
Issued by:

Copy no.
Holder no.
Date   Issue no.

Example 14.3: ***Contents of the Quality Manual***

RTLL : QUALITY MANUAL	Revision no: Issue no: Date:
Section : CONTENTS	Page:
0.0 General 0.1 Amendment sheet 0.2 Distribution list 0.3 Abbreviation 0.4 Definition	
1.0 Introduction 1.1 Purpose of Manual 1.2 Scope of this Manual 1.3 Administration of this manual 1.4 Field of activities	
2.0 Laboratory Quality Policy 2.1 Quality Policy Objective 2.2 Commitment to good professional practices 2.3 Commitment to laboratory's standard of services 2.4 Commitment to compliance to this standard	
3.0 Management requirements 3.1 Organization and management structure 3.2 Laboratory's legal responsibility 3.3 Laboratory's status (Permanent, temporary or mobile) 3.4 Conflict of interest 3.5 Technical management 3.6 Job description of technical manager 3.7 Job description of quality manager 3.8 Job description of chief chemist 3.9 Job description of chemist/analyst 3.10 Job description of quality executive 3.11 Job description of junior chemist/analyst 3.12 Independence of judgement 3.13 Confidentiality and integrity 3.14 Supervision accuracy 3.15 Improper influence 3.16 Confidentiality of clients proprietary rights and information 3.17 Nomination of deputies 3.18 Departure from documented policy and procedures	

RTLL : QUALITY MANUAL	Revision no: Issue no: Date:
Section : CONTENTS	Page:

RTLL : QUALITY MANUAL	Revision no: Issue no: Date:
Section : CONTENTS	Page:

RTLL : QUALITY MANUAL	Revision no: Issue no: Date:
Section : CONTENTS	Page:

RTLL : QUALITY MANUAL	Revision no: Issue no: Date:
Section : CONTENTS	Page:

RTLL : QUALITY MANUAL	Revision no: Issue no: Date:
Section : CONTENTS	Page:

Section 0 : General
0.0 General 0.1 Amendment sheet 0.2 Distribution list 0.3 Abbreviation 0.4 Definition

RTLL : QUALITY MANUAL	Revision no: Issue no: Date:
Section 0: General	Page:

0.0 GENERAL

The test or calibration laboratory shall define its location, head office and the general activities of the laboratory or the company to which it belongs.

(Sample: RTLL is located at Mayur Vihar, New Delhi, India. The laboratory has its head office and work place at the same place. It does not have any other sister concern. The main business of the laboratory is testing of chemical and biological items received from the clients. The laboratory also imparts training and consultancy to the clients for developing quality documentation.)

0.1 AMENDMENT SHEET

The laboratory shall provide the status of Quality Manual and necessary amendments issued be incorporated in the manual. The copy of the amendment shall be sent to the concerned holder of the copy of the Quality Manual. Table 14.1 shows the history of amendments.

Table 14.1: *Amendment history*

Amendment deleted	*Amendment incorporated*
Date: Section: Amendment:	Date: Amendment: Authorized by:

0.2 DISTRIBUTION LIST

0.2.1 Distribution

The laboratory shall explain how and to whom the controlled manual are distributed and maintained. It is also to mention that Xerox copies of Quality Manual are not controlled and marked as "UNCONTROLLED". The name of manual's copy holder should not be included but designation or title of concerned personnel should be used to make it easier to control the manual as individuals might be either transferred or promoted also.

0.2.2 Distribution List

Controlled copies of this manual are printed on special paper and are provided for every manager, quality director and C.E.O. Uncontrolled copies of the manual may be sent to the clients of the laboratory.

Sample

Table 14.2: *Distribution list*

Title	*Department*	*Copy no.*	*Location*
C.E.O.	Head Office	01	Office
Quality Director	Quality department	02	Office
Quality Manager	Quality department	03	Office
Technical Manager	Technical Department	04	Office
Others			

0.3 ABBREVIATIONS

It is observed that many manuals include abbreviations which may not be clearly understood by the reader of the manual. It is also good idea to define these abbreviations.

Sample

C.E.O. — Chief Executive Officer
QSP — Quality System Procedures
SOP — Standard Operating Procedures
Q M — Quality Manager
TM — Technical Manager
e.tc.

0.4 DEFINITIONS

It is observed that laboratories describe certain terms in their Quality Manual. They should be clearly described.

Sample

Test sample: The item received by the laboratory to carry out test, in accordance with specifications, to meet the requirement of client.

Internal Auditor: The test or calibration personnel nominated by the quality manager to conduct internal audit.

0.5 AUTHORIZATION

CEO of RTLL has authorized the quality manager to sign on each page of quality manual and to approve QSP and SOPs and other quality related documentation.

Signature

CEO (RTLL)

Dated:

Section 1 : Introduction to the Manual	
1.0	Introduction
1.1	Purpose of Manual
1.2	Scope of this Manual
1.3	Administration of this manual
1.4	Field of activities

RTLL : QUALITY MANUAL	Revision no: Issue no: Date:
Section 1: Introduction to Manual	Page:

1.0 INTRODUCTION

This Quality Manual is prepared by the laboratory to comply to the requirements of accreditation as laid down in ISO 17025:1999 standard for accreditation of laboratories. The Quality Manual is a document describing the policy and procedure to achieve reliable test or calibration data.

1.1 PURPOSE OF THE MANUAL

The primary purpose of the manual is to develop a general practice to follow the policy and procedures as laid down in the manual. The second purpose of the manual is to implement the requirements of the laboratory quality system and technical competence and to obtain accreditation and to make familiar the test or calibration personnel with the quality system documentation. The laboratory clients should be delighted about the competence and capability of laboratory as reflected through manual.

1.2 SCOPE OF THE MANUAL

This Quality Manual covers the management of the laboratory (You have to describe the management of your laboratory.)

The management of the laboratory includes the management of quality related systems and the personnel directly responsible to conduct test or calibration of samples or items.

Thus a most efficient way to describe the job responsibilities related to quality is to include all of the quality responsibilities in a table format.

Sample

The job responsibilities for implementing and maintaining quality system and technical competence of laboratory are shown in Table 14.3.

Table 14.3: *Job description for quality responsibility*

Title	*Responsibility*	*Reporting to*
CEO Quality Director	Leadership and staffing, technical and quality system, signing test reports	Board of Directors CEO
Technical Manager	Testing, internal calibration, maintenance, interpretation, SOP and QSP writing	Quality Director
Chief Chemist	Testing, calibration, supervision, quality assurance, reference materials, uncertainty of measurement and interpretation, SOP and QSP writing, checking test reports	Technical Manager
Junior Analyst	Analysis, test record maintaining, amendment preparation	Chief Chemist
Quality Manager	Writing Quality Manual, QSP, developing QSP, organizing internal audit, management review, complaint redressel, interpretation, issuing quality documentation, Quality Manual review	CEO and Quality Director
Quality Executive	Writing Quality Manual, QSP, developing records, maintenance of documentation, assisting quality manager.	Quality Manager

1.3 ADMINISTRATION OF THIS MANUAL

Clearly describe how the Quality Manual shall be administered, what is the quality manager's responsibility in implementing and monitoring the Quality Manual, his direct access to highest level of management, role of technical manager, arrangements in absence of key laboratory staff, who are authorized to approve and issue the manual and review and approve changes etc.

1.4 FIELD OF ACTIVITIES

The major field of test or calibration activities undertaken should be spelled out by the laboratory.

Section 2 : Laboratory Quality Policy	
2.0	Laboratory Quality Policy
2.1	Quality Policy Objective
2.2	Commitment to good professional practices
2.3	Commitment to laboratory's standard of services
2.4	Commitment to compliance to this standard

RTLL : QUALITY MANUAL	Revision no: Issue no: Date:
Section 2: Laboratory Quality Policy	Page:

2.0 QUALITY POLICY

The laboratory has to define overall quality intentions and directions of the laboratory as regards to quality.

Sample

"To provide testing and analytical services of recognized standards conforming to specific requirements for pesticides, effluent and water."

2.1 QUALITY POLICY OBJECTIVES

As apart from Quality Policy, the Quality Policy objectives should indicate what is aimed at to achieve.

Sample

The Quality Policy Objectives are compliance to standards, specifications, test or calibration quality improvement, establishment of laboratory's performance and customer's satisfaction.

2.2 COMMITMENT TO GOOD PROFESSIONAL PRACTICES

It should be clearly indicated that the top management is going to ensure and maintain implementation of good professional practices, like adherence to Quality Policy, Quality Policy objectives, quality system procedures with continuous improvement.

2.3 COMMITMENT TO LABORATORY'S STANDARD OF SERVICES

The striving for continuous improvement in laboratory's standard of services should be reflected as matter of integrity and discipline ensured by top management and laboratory personnel.

2.4 COMMITMENT TO COMPLIANCE TO THIS STANDARD

This should be evident from a declaration that the staff are familiar with quality system documentation, Quality Policy and Quality Policy objectives, quality system procedures and their involvement, good faith and discipline, commitment to continuous improvement results in compliance to the high standards of laboratory service upheld by the management.

Section 3 : Management requirements

3.1 Organization and management structure
3.2 Laboratory's legal responsibility
3.3 Laboratory's status (Permanent, temporary or mobile)
3.4 Conflict of interest
3.5 Technical management
3.6 Job description of technical manager
3.7 Job description of quality manager
3.8 Job description of chief chemist
3.9 Job description of chemist/analyst
3.10 Job description of quality executive
3.11 Job description of junior chemist/analyst
3.12 Independence of judgement
3.13 Confidentiality and integrity
3.14 Supervision accuracy
3.15 Improper influence
3.16 Confidentiality of clients, proprietary rights and information
3.17 Nomination of deputies
3.18 Departure from documented policy and procedures

RTLL : QUALITY MANUAL	Revision No. Issue no: Date:
Section 3: Management requirements	Page:

3.1 ORGANIZATION AND MANAGEMENT STRUCTURE

An organization chart clearly describing the position should be developed by the concerned laboratory and roles for various positions should be fixed in a management structure, for example Fig. 14.1 may be referred.

3.2 LABORATORY'S LEGAL RESPONSIBILITY

The legal identity of the laboratory has to be explained so that the clients as well as the laboratory personnel are aware whether it is a registered society, incorporated under the Company's act or a government body.

3.3 LABORATORY'S STATUS — PERMANENT, TEMPORARY OR MOBILE

The laboratory may be operating as a permanent entity or a temporary one, either independently or as an in house unit with in a large company. Some times mobile facilities are set up for access to diverse locations. All units of such nature should be highlighted for the benefit of the users and complying to the accreditation requirements.

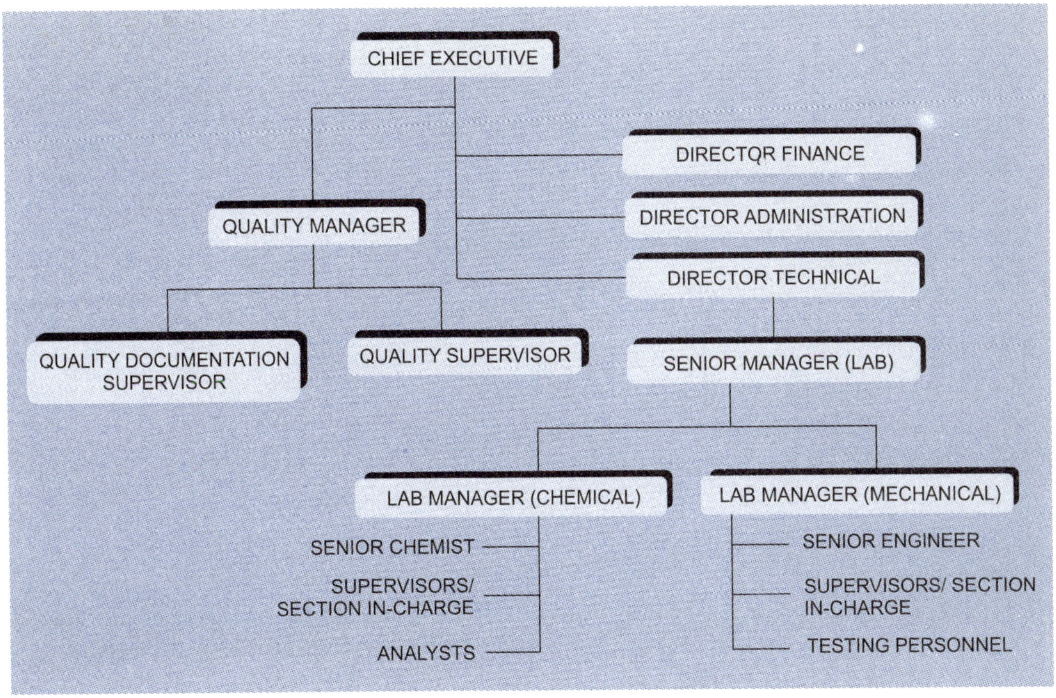

Fig. 14.1: *Operational organization chart of RTLL (ref. sub section 3.1)*

3.4 CONFLICT OF INTEREST

If there is any conflict of interest, by virtue of fields of testing, or between business of the parent company and the laboratory itself, e.g. production activity of parent organization versus testing services of the laboratory or because of clients, requirements or competition with other laboratories, it must be spelled out. Then users and the laboratory personnel can determine their requirements with more clarity and interpret the limitations on results, delivery of reports or confidentiality in this context.

3.5 TECHNICAL MANAGEMENT

The technical management should be clearly identified with fixed job descriptions, preferably tabulated or given as a chart distinctly, so as to avoid any confusion and occasion of indecision.

3.6 JOB DESCRIPTION OF TECHNICAL MANAGER

As covered in Table 14.3 in section 1.

3.7 JOB DESCRIPTION OF CHIEF CHEMIST

As covered in Table 14.3 in section 1.

3.8 JOB DESCRIPTION OF CHEMIST/ANALYST

As covered in Table 14.3 in section 1.

3.9 JOB DESCRIPTION OF QUALITY EXECUTIVE

As covered in Table 14.3 in section 1.

3.10 JOB DESCRIPTION OF JUNIOR CHEMIST/ANALYST

Covered in Table 14.3 in section 1.

3.11 JOB DESCRIPTION OF QUALITY MANAGER

Covered in Table 14.3 in section 1.

3.12 INDEPENDENCE OF JUDGEMENT

A declaration to this effect has to be provided.

Sample Declaration

RTLL test or calibration personnel are free from financial as well as internal or external pressures to give independent judgement regarding the test or calibration results.

3.13 CONFIDENTIALITY AND INTEGRITY

Sample

The test results so obtained are sent only through registered post to the concerned authorized representative of the clients. Any other person is not entertained directly by any laboratory test personnel conducting testing of the sample. A clause has been specially incorporated in the appointment letter of the laboratory personnel to terminate his/her services in case they leak out confidential information to any outsider or if it is established that his/her integrity is doubtful.

3.14 SUPERVISION ADEQUACY

Your laboratory has to ensure adequate supervision and declare it here.

Sample

RTLL shall maintain supervision ratio in a standard form of 1:5 (i.e. one person supervising five persons).

3.15 IMPROPER INFLUENCE

Sample

RTLL follows a confidential system for the samples to be tested or analysed by concerned chemist or analyst. In order to avoid improper influence, client has no direct access to test personnel except the authorized ones in the laboratory.

3.16 CONFIDENTIALITY OF CLIENT'S PROPRIETARY RIGHTS AND INFORMATION

A mechanism to control these aspects should be written.

Sample

RTLL maintains confidentiality of clients proprietary rights through recodification of samples and disclosing the test results only to the authorized representative of the clients.

These results can not be used by any one other than the client or reproduced with out prior permission of laboratory for litigation.

3.17 NOMINATION OF DEPUTIES

Deputy can not be nominated for each test or calibration personnel. Laboratory should think about its capability to manage.

Sample

RTLL has nominated the quality executive to hold quality manager's responsibility in addition to his/her own responsibility in case quality manager is on leave or tour.

3.18 DEPARTURE FROM DOCUMENTED POLICY AND PROCEDURE

Describe your own policy for departure.

Sample

RTLL takes corrective action whenever there is departure from documented policy and procedures in implementing a quality system procedure or standard operating procedures.

Signature
CEO (RTLL)
Dated:

Section 4 : Quality System
4.1 Quality system policies 4.2 Quality system objectives 4.3 Quality system documentation structure 4.4 Reference to quality system documents

RTLL : QUALITY MANUAL	Revision no: Issue no: Date:
Section 4: Quality System	Page:

4.1 QUALITY SYSTEM POLICIES

Define quality system policies, objectives, documentation structure and reference to quality system document.

Sample

RTLL implements and maintains its quality system to comply to the requirements of ISO 17025:1999 with the objective to improve the quality of the test results. RTLL is committed to adopt a four tier quality system to achieve this objective. The four tier quality system includes –

Level 1: Quality Manual
Level 2: Quality System Procedures
Level 3: Standard Operating Procedures
Level 4: Quality Records

4.2 QUALITY SYSTEM OBJECTIVES

The objective of quality system related to test or calibration should be given.

4.3 QUALITY SYSTEM DOCUMENTATION STRUCTURE

Describe quality system documentation structure.

Sample

RTLL is committed to follow four tier quality system documentation structure to achieve the objective of quality policy.

4.4 REFERENCE TO QUALITY SYSTEM DOCUMENTS

Provide reference to quality system documents wherever it is necessary.

Sample

Reference to standard operating procedures or quality system procedure may be given in relation with accreditation elements.

Signature
CEO (RTLL)
Date

Section 5 : Document Control	
5.1	Document approval and issue
5.2	Document control procedures
5.3	Document change and control in computerized documentation
5.4	Document identification

RTLL : QUALITY MANUAL	Revision no: Issue no: Date:
Section 5 : Document Control	Page:

5. 0 DOCUMENT CONTROL

This section requires that you specify how the documents are controlled. (i.e who approves and issues what documents and how are they updated.)

Sample

Authorization requirements vary and are documented either in a document or in a procedure controlling it. Individuals receiving controlled document are responsible to ensure that they replace the obsolete copy with new one. Documents are reviewed on need basis. The following Table – 14.4 describes the controlled documents, who issues them and how are they controlled.

Table 14.4: *Controlled documents*

Quality Document	*Issued by*	*Controlled by*
Quality Manual	Quality Manager	Doc. Control
Quality System Procedure	Quality Manager	Doc. Control
Quality System Procedure	Quality Manager	Doc. Control
Standard Operating Procedures	Quality Manager	Doc. Control
Test Reports	Quality Manager	Doc. Control
Internal Audit	Quality Manager	Doc. Control
Management Review	Quality Manager	Doc. Control
Tender and Contract Reviews	Technical Manager	Doc. Control

5.1 DOCUMENT APPROVAL AND ISSUE

State here who approves the quality documentation and who is authorized by the top management to sign on each page of Quality Manual, Standard Operating Procedures and Quality System Procedure and to issue the quality documentation.

Sample

CEO of RTLL approves the quality documentation and authorizes quality manager to sign on each page of the manual, quality procedures and standard operating procedures and to issue the same to concerned.

5.2 DOCUMENT CONTROL PROCEDURES

The laboratory may adopt a numbering system for various quality documents and records. For example, QSP 501: Procedure for identification and numbering the documents.

5.3 DOCUMENT CHANGE, REVIEW AND REAFFIRMATION

It should be described how and why the changes are made in document. A quality procedure may be evolved by the laboratory.

For example, QSP 502: Procedure for preparation, issue and control of new documents/amendments to existing documents.

5.4 DOCUMENT CHANGE AND CONTROL IN COMPUTERIZED DOCUMENTATION

When there is quality documentation on computer, attempt has to be made by the laboratory to formulate a quality procedure for control of computerized quality documentation.

Sample

RTLL controls the computerized quality documentation through an identification and numbering system for various quality documents. Prior to any change to be made in a document, the earlier script matter is retained on computer or hard copy is kept for reference.

For example, QSP 503: Procedure for control of computerized quality documentation.

5.5 DOCUMENT IDENTIFICATION

There has to be an easier process for identifying quality documents supervision, checking of test report/calibration certificates, internal/external audit, and management review. Now it is to be decided how and what corrective action is to be taken for nonconforming work related to quality system and technical operations.

Sample

RTLL identifies its documents through suffix of the documents. Such as

QSP: Quality System Procedures
SOP: Standard Operating Procedures
IP: Indian Pharmacopoeia
BP: British Pharmacopoeia
SP: Specification
CC: Calibration Certificate
TR: Test Request

Section 6 : Review of request, tender and contract
6.1 Client's test request and tender for item testing 6.2 Review of request and tender 6.3 Review of contract 6.4 Communication to client 6.5 Records of reviews

RTLL : QUALITY MANUAL	Revision no: Issue no: Date:
Section 6: Review of request, tender and contract	Page:

6.0 REVIEW OF REQUEST, TENDER AND CONTRACT

The laboratory is required to make a procedure to review test request, tender and contract for testing.

Samples

6.1 Client's test request and tender are identified by laboratory identification system on receipt.

6.2 The test requests received from the clients are reviewed for selection of test methods wherever test methods are not described by the clients. On selection of the test method, communication is sent to the client for his comment and confirmation.

6.3 Tender and contract are reviewed to resolve any differing requirement mentioned in the tender of the clients. Communication is made, regarding reviews of contracts, to the clients and records of such reviews are maintained by the laboratory.

6.4 Records are retained for a specified period till the final settlement of contract of testing or calibration is completed.

For example, QSP 601 Procedure for test request, tender and contract review, may be referred.

Section 7 : Subcontracting of testing

RTLL : QUALITY MANUAL	Revision no: Issue no: Date:
Section 7: Subcontracting of Testing	Page:

7.0 SUBCONTRACTING OF TESTING

Laboratory's policy for subcontracting work should be declared. If there is no subcontracting of testing of items to test laboratories then a statement may be made that "The laboratory does not carry out subcontracting of testing items". If there is any subcontracting of testing items then the laboratory will have to spell that out.

Sample

Presently RTLL is not involved in subcontracting of testing however if need arises it shall be done with the test laboratories complying to the requirements of ISO 17025:1999. The records of such subcontracted laboratories shall be maintained and made available whenever required by concerned national regulation body.

For Example, QSP 701: Procedure for selection of subcontracting of test laboratories, may be referred.

Section 8 : Purchasing services and supplies	
8.1	Selection of purchase services and supplies
8.2	Compliance of the supplied consumables to specifications
8.3	Purchase order and review
8.4	Supplier's evaluation for critical consumables
8.5	Records of suppliers

RTLL : QUALITY MANUAL	Revision no: Issue no: Date:
Section 8: Purchasing services and supplies	Page:

8.0 PURCHASING SERVICES AND SUPPLIES

Laboratory policy and procedure have to be spelled out for this and persons responsible for implementing have to be designated so.

Sample

8.1 RTLL shall use the services of qualified suppliers for consumables, equipment procurement, their maintenance and calibration. Selection of suppliers shall be made in accordance with their capability to comply with terms and conditions of the purchase contract.

8.2 The purchased items, consumables etc. shall be verified for compliance to specifications. RTLL shall maintain records of such verifications.

8.3 Purchase order shall be reviewed for incorporating new requirements if any.

8.4 Suppliers of critical consumables shall be evaluated in accordance with vendors' specifications available in the country.

8.5 RTLL shall maintain records of such suppliers.

Ref: QSP 801: Procedure for selection and evaluation of suppliers' services to laboratories.

Section 9 : Service to the client
9.1 Access of the client to the laboratory 9.2 Witnessing of test by the client 9.3 Communication to the client 9.4 Other feedback from the client

RTLL : QUALITY MANUAL	Revision no: Issue no: Date:
Section 9: Service to the client	Page:

9.0 SERVICE TO THE CLIENT

Your laboratory has to include a paragraph for the policy followed. Laboratory personnel responsible to authorize the customers for these services should be identified, if required.

Sample

9.1 and 9.2 RTLL shall provide access to its clients to witness the tests if any doubt occurs regarding the performance of the test or specific test. (Ref. LQSP no. ....).

9.3 RTLL shall communicate to the client about the delay in testing of large contractual assignments. (Ref. LQSP no. ....).

9.4 RTLL shall collect feedback for continuous improvement in its quality system from its clients for performing its services and cooperation, and refer to records maintained (Ref. LQSP no. ....) for the lessons learnt.

Section 10 : Complaints
10.1 Complaint redressel procedure 10.2 Investigation against complaint 10.3 Complaints record

RTLL : QUALITY MANUAL	Revision no: Issue no: Date:
Section 10: Complaints	Page:

10. Complaint

Spell out policy for complaints and how would you identify and resolve internal or external nontechnical or technical complaints.

Sample

10.1 RTLL shall identify the persons responsible for resolution of complaint, identify the complaint, record it in its register for resolving on priority through a complaint redressel procedure.

10.2 RTLL shall initiate step wise investigation by assigning the responsibility to a qualified and experienced internal auditor.

10.3 RTLL shall maintain records of complaints redressel.

Ref. QSP 1001: Procedure for complaints redressel.

Section 11 : Policy for control of nonconforming testing or calibration work
11.1 Management of nonconforming work 11.2 Evaluation of nonconforming work 11.3 Responsibility for resumption of nonconforming work 11.4 Corrective action for recurring nonconforming work

RTLL : QUALITY MANUAL	Revision no: Issue no: Date:
Section 11: Policy for control of nonconforming testing or calibration work	Page:

11. POLICY FOR CONTROL OF NONCONFORMING TESTING OR CALIBRATION WORK

With what and how you proceed if there is nonconforming test or calibration work, should be mentioned.

Sample

11.1 RTLL shall withhold further processing of testing or calibration of items or samples in case the procedure followed is not in conformity with documented procedure. The nonconforming work shall be identified and responsibility to manage the same shall be assigned either to quality manager, technical manager or chief chemist depending upon the nature of nonconforming work.

11.2 Nonconforming work related to quality system and technical operation of laboratory shall be reviewed to take prompt action to evaluate significance of nonconforming work to arrive on a decision for its acceptability on corrections.

11.2.1 RTLL shall recall the nonconforming work from clients on its identification.

11.3 Quality Director shall be responsible to authorize quality manager or technical manager for resumption of nonconforming work or necessary corrections.

11.4 RTLL shall follow quarterly corrective action for recurring nonconforming work. The records of such corrective actions are maintained.

Ref: QSP 1101: Procedure for identification of nonconforming work related to quality system and technical operation.

Section 12 : Corrective action
12.1 Authority to implement corrective action 12.2 Cause analysis 12.3 Selection and implementation of corrective action 12.4 Monitoring of corrective action 12.5 Additional audit for noncomplying activity

RTLL : QUALITY MANUAL	Revision no: Issue no: Date:
Section 12: Corrective Action	Page:

12. CORRECTIVE ACTION

The evidence of unsatisfactory quality related to quality system, technical operation or services may be available from many sources like customer's complaints or quality control. Instrument calibration, consumables checking, staff's observations or supervision, checking out the test reports/calibration certificate, internal/external audit or management review. Now it needs to be decided what is policy, what corrective action is taken and how, for the nonconforming work related to quality system and technical operations. It also needs to be determined that what type of problem shall have to be brought out by whom and what quality system procedures shall be referred for corrective action (Table 14.5).

Sample

Table 14.5: *Corrective actions*

Type of problem	*Discovered by*	*Corrective action*
Customer's complaints	Client	See QSP
Quality Control	Technical Manager	See QSP
Instrument Calibration	Supervisor	See QSP
Consumables Checking	Supervisor	See SOP
Staff's observation/supervision	Staff	See records
Checking of test report or calibration certificate	Supervisor	See records
Internal/external Audit	Auditors	See records
Management Review	Quality Manager	See records

12.1 CEO of RTLL shall authorize the Quality Director to implement corrective actions for nonconforming work related to quality system and technical operations. The implementation of the same shall be substantiated by documentary evidences.

12.2 RTLL shall identify the potential causes of unsatisfactory quality of test through examination of clients' requirements, samples specification, method and procedures, staff skill/competence training, consumables quality, equipment calibration status for developing appropriate corrective action.

12.3 RTLL shall identify, select and implement potential corrective action to eliminate the recurrence of the problem. RTLL shall record any change resulting from corrective action.

12.4 and 12.5 Corrective actions implemented for recurring problems related to quality system and technical operations shall be periodically monitored and if necessary an additional internal audit shall be carried out on doubts for nonconformance to standard requirements.

Ref: QSP 1201 – Procedure for determining potential cause for corrective action.

Section 13 : Preventive action
13.1 Identification of sources of preventive action 13.2 Preventive action plan 13.3 Preventive Action Procedure 13.4 Preventive action record

RTLL : QUALITY MANUAL	Revision no: Issue no: Date:
Section 13: Preventive Action	Page:

13 PREVENTIVE ACTION

State the policy on preventive actions for required improvements and tracing out where and when a preventive action may be taken.

13.1 and 13.2 RTLL shall identify and authorize laboratory personnel, identify potential sources of nonconformance related to quality system and technical operations and develop plans for preventive action and monitor the same for further improvement.

13.3 and 13.4 RTLL shall develop procedure of preventive action control nonconformance related to quality system and technical operation. Records shall be maintained for the preventive action taken.

Ref. QSP 1301: Procedure for preventive action for analysis of data, trend, risk analysis and inter-laboratory comparison, and maintenance of records.

Section 14 : Control of Records

RTLL : QUALITY MANUAL	Revision no: Issue no: Date:
Section 14: Control of Records	Page:

14.0 CONTROL OF RECORDS

The policy to maintain the records and their control should be described.

One of the easiest ways, to address the procedures involved and identification of the persons responsible, is the table format.

Sample

Table 14.6: *Control of quality records*

Records	*Purpose*	*Owner*	*Location*	*Retention*
Equipment maintenance	Equipment history	Maintenance Supervisor	Maintenance Section	5 years
Raw data	Calculation	Supervisor	Chemical Laboratory	3 years
Calibration certificate	Equipment performance	Supervisor	Chemical Laboratory	5 years

RTLL shall implement and maintain a procedure to identify, storage, security, indexing, access, retention, dispositions and correction in records.

Ref. QSP 1401: Procedure for control of records.

Section 15 : Internal audits
15.1 Internal audit plan 15.2 Internal auditor's qualification and training 15.3 Internal audit periodicity 15.4 Record of audit findings 15.5 Record of corrective action for audit findings 15.6 Follow up action on audit record

RTLL : QUALITY MANUAL	Revision no: Issue no: Date:
Section 15: Internal Audit	Page:

15 INTERNAL AUDITS

Briefly state the policy, who will conduct internal audit and how often and who will be informed of the audit.

Sample

RTLL quality manager shall plan and organize quarterly internal audits related to quality system and technical operations by nominating qualified, trained and experienced persons as auditors. The audit findings shall be reported to quality manager. The corrective action shall be taken for audit findings by the concerned personnel, which shall be verified by the quality manager. The records of internal audit, corrective and follow up action shall be maintained.

Ref: QSP 1501: Procedure to conduct internal audits, and
QSP 1502: Procedure for internal audit plan and scheduling

Section 16 : Management review
16.1 Periodicity of review 16.2 Records of review 16.3 Follow-up of review decision

RTLL : QUALITY MANUAL	Revision no: Issue no: Date:
Section 16: Management Review	Page:

16. MANAGEMENT REVIEW

Describe the management review policy including, how often the quality systems and technical operations related to laboratory are reviewed, and scope of activities to be reviewed, and persons responsible for holding the review. Describe the procedure of management review.

Sample

CEO, RTLL shall nominate members of a management review committee. The quality manager shall plan and organize yearly review of quality system and technical operation related to chemical and microbiological laboratory. The review shall cover the nonconforming work related to quality system and technical operation, findings of internal/external audits, and clients' complaints. The follow up action shall be taken on review findings by the concerned staff and *records* (*refer to record documents*) of reviews and follow-up action on reviews shall be maintained and made available on demands.

Ref: QSP 1601: Procedure for nominating members of management review committee, and

QSP 1602: Procedure to conduct Management Review

Section 17 : Technical requirements
17.1 General factors for correctness and reliability of test or calibration 17.2 Specific factors affecting test or calibration reliability

RTLL : QUALITY MANUAL	Revision no: Issue no: Date:
Section 17: Technical Requirements	Page:

17. TECHNICAL REQUIREMENTS

Describe what are general and specific technical factors affecting the correctness and reliability of the test data.

Sample

RTLL shall identify the general and specific factors affecting the correctness and reliability of test or calibration. RTLL shall also identify the specific factors contributing to the total uncertainty of measurement.

Ref. 1701: Procedure to identify factors affecting the quality and reliability of test data.

Section 18 : Personnel

RTLL : QUALITY MANUAL	Revision no: Issue no: Date:
Section 18: Personnel	Page:

18. PERSONNEL

Apart from stating the policy for maintaining personnel competence, answers are needed to following questions –

What type of technical personnel are employed, do they meet the qualification and experience requirements of relevant specific criteria. How on the job training is provided to test personnel on transferring them to other type of testing. Goals regarding the training of personnel should be set.

Sample

18.1 RTLL shall employ test personnel having appropriate qualification and experience in the areas related to chemical or microbiological testing.

18.1.1 RTLL shall employ internal calibration personnel having appropriate qualification, experience and training in instruments calibration related to chemical or microbiological testing.

18.2 The internal or external training needs shall be identified and be provided to test or internal calibration personnel if deemed necessary. Records of such training shall be maintained and retained.

18.3 RTLL does not employ contracted test or calibration personnel however if necessary they shall be allowed to perform testing of samples in case they comply to the requirements of education, experience and on job trainings as prescribed by relevant specific criteria.

18.3.1 The contractual personnel shall be supervised by the permanently employed supervisors of RTLL.

18.4 Job description shall be as per Table no. 14.3.

18.5, 18.6 and 18.7 RTLL shall authorize the test personnel to operate sophisticated instruments and prepare, sign test reports, and to issue the same to the clients. The records of such authorization shall be maintained.

Ref: QSP 1801: Procedure for identification of training needs, and
QSP 1802: Procedure for on job training

Section 19 : Accommodation and environmental conditions

RTLL : QUALITY MANUAL	Revision no: Issue no: Date:
Section 19: Accommodation and Environmental Conditions	Page:

19. ACCOMMODATION AND ENVIRONMENTAL CONDITIONS

Here describe the policy, and design of laboratory and its suitability to testing or calibration of items, environmental control, availability of facilities, control of access to restricted areas of laboratory, so as to facilitate the required performance of test or calibration.

Sample

19.1 and 19.2 RTLL is having the appropriate design of laboratory. The lay out of instrument, equipments are suitable to carry out tests and specific tests of chemical and microbiological nature on samples. RTLL shall maintain appropriate test conditions complying to specifications to produce reliable test or calibration results.

19.3 and 19.4 The laboratory environment shall be duly monitored and recorded by the qualified supervisors. *(refer to record documentation.)*

19.5 and 19.6 The RTLL shall control the cross contamination through appropriate checks and control mechanism. The access of clients and laboratory personnel shall be restricted to areas where hazardous chemical or biological samples are tested.

19.7 RTLL shall maintain good house keeping and also comply to national safety regulations applicable to testing of hazardous chemicals.

Ref. QSP 1901: Procedure for environment control and monitoring, and
QSP 1902: Procedure for good house keeping, and
QSP 1903: Procedure for safety regulations

Section 20 : Test or calibration method and method validation
20.1 Standard method 20.2 Selection of methods 20.3 Communication to client for use of selected method 20.4 Method developed by laboratory 20.5 Nonstandard method 20.6 Agreement with client for use of nonstandard method 20.7 Validation of methods 20.8 Method validation procedures 20.9 Records of validation of methods

RTLL : QUALITY MANUAL	Revision no: Issue no: Date:
Section 20: Test or Calibration Method and Method Validation	Page:

20. TEST AND CALIBRATION METHOD AND METHOD VALIDATION

State the relevant policy and explain whether your laboratory has adopted test or calibration methods stipulated in national or international specifications, pharmacopoeias, or text books. If your laboratory uses self designed, client's, nonstandard or modified test or calibration method than VALIDATE them before actually putting into practice.

Sample

20.1, 20.4 and 20.5 RTLL shall use standard test or calibration methods described in the national or international specifications, text books or pharmacopoeias but when ever necessary it shall use validated laboratory developed method, clients' method or a nonstandard method for testing or internal calibration of samples or items.

20.2 and 20.3 RTLL shall select test methods whenever these are not mentioned in the test request of clients and communicate to the clients its use in sample analysis.

20.5 and 20.6 RTLL shall have an agreement with the clients for use of their method or nonstandard method. Validation of the method shall be confirmed prior to its use by RTLL.

20.7 Wherever necessary RTLL shall validate self designed, modified or nonstandard test methods.

20.8 and 20.9 RTLL shall follow appropriate method validation procedure and records of such validations shall be maintained.

Ref. QSP 2001: Procedure for selection of test methods when client has not mentioned the method, and

QSP 2002: Procedure for method validations

SOP 2001: Standard operating procedures for chemical testing of samples

SOP 2002: Standard operating procedures for microbiological testing of samples

Section 21 : Estimation of uncertainty of measurement
21.1 Internal calibration's uncertainty of measurement 21.2 Identification of component of uncertainty for specific cases 21.3 Methods of analysis of uncertainty 21.4 Records of uncertainty of measurement

RTLL : QUALITY MANUAL	Revision no: Issue no: Date:
Section 21: Estimation of Uncertainty of Measurement	Page:

21. ESTIMATION OF UNCERTAINTY OF MEASUREMENT

Uncertainty of measurement is required by most of the laboratories involved in calibration of instrument or equipments but some times it can be required by a client also, for some specific test.

Sample

21.1 and 21.2 RTLL shall estimate the uncertainty of measurement for internal calibration of instruments or equipments, and specific tests. The components of uncertainty of measurement have been identified for calculation purpose.

21.3 and 21.4 RTLL shall adopt appropriate method for calculation of uncertainty of measurement and records of the same shall be maintained.

Ref. QSP 2101: Procedure for determining uncertainty of measurements.

Section 22 : Control of data
22.1 Checks on data transfer 22.2 Use of computer for data 22.3 Validation of computer software 22.4 Procedure for data protection and confidentiality

RTLL : QUALITY MANUAL	Revision no: Issue no: Date:
Section 22: Control of Data	Page:

22. CONTROL OF DATA

Explain what checks you have used to control the data transfer in your laboratory.

Sample

22.1 RTLL shall check the data prior to transfer to permanent records. The checked data shall be signed by concerned supervisor.

22.2 and 22.3 The computer software used for collecting, transferring and correcting data shall be periodically validated and records of such validations shall be maintained and retained for appropriate period.

22.4 RTLL shall use pass words and allow authorized personnel only to use computers for data development.

Ref. QSP 2201: Procedure for security of computerized data.

Section 23 : Equipment	
23.1	Use of equipment outside permanent control
23.2	Accuracy compliance of equipment and software with test specification
23.3	Calibration programme for key items of equipment
23.4	Authorization of personnel for operation and maintenance of equipment
23.5	Identification of equipment and software items
23.6	Equipment's safe handling, transport and storage
23.7	Equipment's maintenance planning
23.8	Identification and labeling of defective equipment
23.9	Equipment's calibration status and labeling
23.10	Equipment's calibration checks before use
23.11	Intermediate calibration checks and records
23.12	Calibration copies' correction
23.13	Equipment and software records
23.14	Equipment's safety from adjustment

RTLL : QUALITY MANUAL	Revision no: Issue no: Date:
Section 23: Equipment	Page:

23. EQUIPMENT

If such equipments are in use which are not under direct control of laboratory, then the policy in use should be stated. Do you have a log book for equipment details? If not, then the same should be developed. If you carry out the maintenance of instrumentation, then very definitely you should be having the procedures too. How do you ensure calibration of instruments/equipments used in testing. Follow practices of legible labeling of calibration status on your instrumentation if not done so far.

Sample

23.1 RTLL shall use instruments for testing of samples which are under its direct control however if need arises, the instruments/equipments of specific nature and appropriate accuracy available with its site division may be used for specific testing. Records for all major test or calibration equipments shall be maintained (refer to the record document.

23.2 RTLL shall use equipment and software of appropriate accuracy complying to the requirements of method being adopted for testing a sample.

23.3 RTLL shall implement and maintain calibration programme for key items of instruments/equipment in case these items affect the test results.

23.4 RTLL's equipments/instruments shall be operated and repaired and calibrated by authorized personnel.

23.5 RTLL shall identify and provide unique numbers to items and software of equipment.

23.6 RTLL shall handle carefully the equipment during transit and maintain the storage of these while complying with the manufacturer's instructions.

23.7 RTLL shall identify and give appropriate numbers to defective equipment and label the equipment as "Out of Order".

23.8 RTLL shall follow preventive and corrective maintenance planning and scheduling for instrumentation to avoid deterioration.

23.9 RTLL shall use labeling for indicating instrument calibration status.

23.10 and 23.11 RTLL shall ensure calibration of such equipment before use which remains outside the direct control of laboratory, however, where the internal calibration checks are followed for ensuring calibration status, it shall be done complying to appropriate procedure.

23.12 RTLL shall use appropriate procedure for correcting calibration copies for updating computer software.

23.13 RTLL shall ensure safeguards of testing, measuring equipments and software from adjustments.

Ref. QSP 2301: Procedure for calibration programme of equipment
QSP 2302: Procedure for numbering of equipment and their software
QSP 2303: Procedure for maintenance planning and scheduling
QSP 2304: Procedure for authorization to operate equipment and to carry out maintenance

Section 24 : Measurement traceability

24.1 Equipment calibration programme
24.2 Traceability to SI units
24.3 Measurement uncertainty in calibration certificate
24.4 Compliance statement to metrological specification
24.5 Traceability to non SI units
24.6 Participation in inter-laboratory comparison

RTLL : QUALITY MANUAL	Revision no: Issue no: Date:
Section 24: Measurement Traceability	Page:

24. MEASUREMENT TRACEABILITY (CALIBRATION)

All measurements or comparisons should be traceable to national or international metrological institutions. Do you follow this practice? If not then start. Formulate and declare the policy, document the procedures established and maintained, identify persons responsible for implementing the same, generate records and provide reference to the document.

Sample

24.1 RTLL shall implement and maintain a calibration programme for its instruments being used for testing of samples related to chemical or microbiological areas.

24.2 The comparisons or measurements made by RTLL shall be traceable to SI units of measurement applicable to primary standards maintained by national or international metrological institutions.

24.3 RTLL shall ensure that all internal calibration certification have mention of uncertainty of measurement, appropriate metrological specifications no., and are traceable to national standard.

24.4 The calibration certification of an equipment obtained from an external calibration laboratory shall be accepted by RTLL in case it has mentioning of uncertainty to national or international metrological institution.

24.5 and 24.6 RTLL shall ensure traceability of comparisons or calibrations to certified reference material or inter-laboratory comparisons where traceability to SI units is not possible.

Ref: QSP 2401: Procedure for calibration traceability

Section 25 : Measurement Traceability (Testing)
25.1 Test measurement traceability to SI units 25.2 Uncertainty of measurement for testing 25.3 Test measurement traceability to non SI units

RTLL : QUALITY MANUAL	Revision no: Issue no: Date:
Section 25: Measurement Traceability (Testing)	Page:

25. MEASUREMENT TRACEABILITY (TESTING)

Measurement related to analysis or testing of samples should have appropriate traceability. A test laboratory should mention its policy, how does it maintain its traceability of test measurement, and identifies the persons responsible.

Sample

25.1 and 25.2 RTLL shall maintain test measurement's traceability to SI units of national or international standard. RTLL shall calculate uncertainty of test measurement if required by a client or as essential requirement of a test. *(Refer to the records generated).*

25.3 RTLL shall ensure traceability of test measurement to certified material or inter-laboratory comparisons where traceability to SI units is not possible.

Section 26 : Reference standard and reference material
26.1 Calibration programme for reference standards 26.2 Calibration traceability for reference standards 26.3 Calibration of reference standard on adjustment 26.4 Reference material traceability to SI units or CRM 26.5 Intermediate checks for reference standard or reference material or SRM 26.6 Transport and storage of reference standard or material

RTLL : QUALITY MANUAL	Revision no: Issue no: Date:
Section 26: Reference Standard and Reference Material	Page:

26. REFERENCE STANDARD AND REFERENCE MATERIAL

Here explain how does your laboratory implement and maintain calibration programme for reference standards or reference materials. Whether they are traceable to a national or international body?

Sample

26.1 and 26.2 RTLL shall plan, implement and maintain a calibration programme for its reference standards accompanied with a certificate traceable to national or international body.

26.3 RTLL shall use reference standard for calibration of equipments. RTLL shall also ensure calibration of reference standard on adjustment, if made any.

26.4 RTLL shall ensure traceability of reference materials to SI units or certified reference material.

26.5 RTLL shall ensure follow up of intermediate checks of calibration status of reference standard, reference material or standard reference material.

26.6 RTLL shall ensure safe handling, storage, and transport of reference standard or reference material.

Ref: QSP 2601: Identification of reference standard and reference material.
QSP 2602: Procedure for safe handling, storage, transport of reference standard or reference material.

Section 27 : Sampling

RTLL : QUALITY MANUAL	Revision no: Issue no: Date:
Section 27: Sampling	Page:

27. SAMPLING

Describe whether the test or calibration laboratory is involved in sampling prior to test or calibration of items or samples. If sampling is a part of testing then state sampling plan, procedures, acceptance and rejection criteria.

Sample

27.1 and 27.2 RTLL being an independent testing laboratory does not carry out any sampling prior to testing however if need arises for a specific testing, appropriate sampling procedure having acceptance and rejection criteria shall be followed. RTLL shall follow modified sampling plans on demand of customers.

27.3 RTLL shall maintain records of sampling procedure which includes sampling procedure number, sample size and identification, environmental condition and sampling location.

Ref: QSP 2701: Sampling procedure writing, approval and implementation.

Section 28 : Handling of test and calibration items
28.1 Transportation procedure 28.2 Sample receipt procedure 28.3 Sample handling procedure 28.4 Sample protection and storage 28.5 Sample retention and disposal 28.6 Sample identification 28.7 Abnormality recording of test or calibration item on receipt 28.8 Sample handling instruction 28.9 Security and storage of secured items

RTLL : QUALITY MANUAL	Revision no: Issue no: Date:
Section 28: Handling of Test and Calibration Items	Page:

28. HANDLING OF TEST AND CALIBRATION ITEMS

Explain how does your laboratory receive samples of testing or calibration from clients. Whether the sample is examined for appropriateness and codified or conditioned in specific environment during storage prior to assigning it to the analyst for carrying out requisite tests. What is your policy on these aspects?

Sample

28.1, 28.2,28.3, 28.4 and 28.5 RTLL shall ensure safe transportation, handling, receipt, storage, protection, retention and disposal of items or samples received from its clients for testing or specific testing.

28.6 RTLL shall provide code number on examination of appropriateness of samples or items to specifications. The code shall be retained on items or samples during various operations inside the chemical or microbiological laboratories. History of handling shall be recorded. *(Refer to the records document).*

28.7 RTLL shall communicate to clients in case the samples or items do not meet the requirements of specification and testing shall be resumed on clarifications from the clients.

28.8 RTLL shall ensure use of appropriate facilities to control the damage or deterioration of items or samples during handling, storage, and sample preparation. RTLL shall maintain and monitor environmental conditions in case items or samples need to be conditioned prior to testing or internal calibration.

28.9 RTLL shall ensure safe and secure storage of items if it is the requirement of specification.

Ref: QSP 2801: Procedure for codification of samples
QSP 2802: Procedure for storage and conditioning of samples
QSP 2803: Procedure for disposal of samples

Section 29 : Assuring the quality of test and calibration
29.1 Quality control for validity of test or calibration 29.2 Use of SQC techniques 29.3 Use of CRM or SRM 29.4 Replicate test by same or different method 29.5 Retest or re-calibration of items 29.6 Correlation of results for different characteristics of items 29.7 Proficiency Testing

RTLL : QUALITY MANUAL	Revision no: Issue no: Date:
Section 29: Assuring the Quality of Test and Calibration	Page:

29. ASSURING THE QUALITY OF TEST AND CALIBRATION

Explain how do you control the quality of testing or calibration of samples or test items in your laboratory. Formulate and declare the policy.

Sample

RTLL shall assure and maintain the quality of testing or calibration results through use of Certified Reference Materials, verification techniques, Statistical Quality Control techniques, repeat analysis, follow up of different methods, co-relations of results for different characteristics of items, inter-laboratory comparisons and Proficiency Testing. Persons responsible shall be designated accordingly and records for all verification practices including inter-laboratory comparisons and/or Proficiency Testing shall be maintained *(Refer to records documentation)*.

Ref: QSP 2901: Procedure for use of control charts
QSP 2902: Procedure for the use of regression analysis for verification of results

Section 30 : Reporting of results

RTLL : QUALITY MANUAL	Revision no: Issue no: Date:
Section 30: Reporting of Results	Page:

30. REPORTING OF RESULTS

State the policy regarding the reporting of results. Identify who will prepare test report, check and sign the test report. Describe what type of test report format for internal or external purpose is used by your laboratory.

Sample

30.1 and 30.2 RTLL shall use approved test report format complying to the requirements of this standard for issuing test results to its clients.

30.3 RTLL shall provide additional information in test reports for interpretation of deviation, exclusion from test, test conditions statement of compliance to specification and uncertainty of measurement.

30.4 and 30.5 For necessary interpretation of calibration results, RTLL shall provide information of environmental conditions of calibration, uncertainty of measurement, statement of compliance to specification and traceability to national or international standard of measurement.

(Note: RTLL does not deal with issuance of calibration certificate to external clients, but regarding internal calibration results it is making this statement.)

30.6 RTLL shall have record of calibration prior and after the adjustments.

30.7 RTLL shall not accept any calibration certificate from a calibration laboratory who has made recommendation for calibration interval of equipment on certificate.

30.8 RTLL shall not give its opinion regarding compliance of test data to specifications or clients requirements.

30.9 The test or calibration reports of RTLL shall clearly mention the test or calibration results obtained from subcontracted laboratories.

30.10 RTLL shall use electronic media to transmit test results to clients on demand. The hard copy of test report shall be sent to client later on.

30.11 RTLL shall use duly designed, approved test or calibration reports complying to the standard. Supplementary test report shall be issued in case of amendments to the test results.

Appendices

Appendix 1

Cross References for Items/ Clauses of ISO/IEC 17025 and ISO/IEC Guide 25

Item from contents list of ISO/IEC 17025	*Clause ISO/IEC 17025*	*Clause ISO/IEC Guide25*
Scope	1.1	1.1
	1.2	N
	1.3	N
	1.4	1.3
	1.5	*7.6 Note*
	1.6	*Intro*
Normative references	2	2
Terms and definitions	3	3
Management requirements		
Organization	4.1.1	4.1
	4.1.2	1.2
	4.1.3	4.1
	4.1.4	N
	4.1.5 (a)	4.2 a)
	4.1.5 (b)	4.2 b)
	4.1.5 (c)	4.2 i)
	4.1.5 (d)	4.2 c)
	4.1.5 (e)	5.2 b), 5.2 c)
	4.1.5 (f)	4.2 d)
	4.1.5 (g)	4.2 e)
	4.1.5 (h)	4.2 f)
	4.1.5 (i)	4.2 g)
	4.1.5 (j)	4.2 h)

Item from contents list of ISO/IEC 17025	*Clause ISO/IEC 17025*	*Clause ISO/IEC Guide25*
Quality system	4.2.1	5.1, 5.4.2
	4.2.2	5.1, 5.2 a)
	4.2.2 (a)	5.1
	4.2.2 (b)	5.2a)
	4.2.2 (c)	5.2 a)
	4.2.2 (d)	5.1
	4.2.2 (e)	5.2
	4.2.3	5.2 m)
	4.2.4	5.2 e)
Document control	4.3.1	5.2 d)
	4.3.2.1	5.2 d)
	4.3.2.2 (a)	5.1, 5.2 d)
	4.3.2.2 (b)	5.2 d)
	4.3.2.2 (c)	5.2 d)
	4.3.2.2 (d)	5.2 d)
	4.3.2.3	5.2 d)
	4.3.3.1	5.2 d)
	4.3.3.2	5.2 d)
	4.3.3.3	5.2 d)
	4.3.3.4	5.2 d)
Review of requests, tenders and contracts	4.4.1	5.2 i)
	4.4.1 (a)	5.2 i)
	4.4.1 (b)	5.2 i)
	4.4.1 (c)	5.2 i)
	4.4.2	5.2 i)
	4.4.3	5.2 i)
	4.4.4	5.2 i)
	4.4.5	5.2 i)
Subcontracting of tests and calibrations	4.5.1	14.1
	4.5.2	14.1
	4.5.3	N
	4.5.4	14.2
Purchasing services and supplies	4.6.1	10.8, 15.2
	4.6.2	15.1
	4.6.3	N
	4.6.4	15.3
Service to the client	4.7	N
Complaints	4.8	16.1
Control of non-conforming work	4.9.1	5.2 o)
	4.9.1 (a)	5.2 o)

Item from contents list of ISO/IEC 17025	*Clause ISO/IEC 17025*	*Clause ISO/IEC Guide25*
	4.9.1 (b)	5.2 o)
	4.9.1 (c)	5.2 o)
	4.9.1 (d)	5.2 o), 13.6
	4.9.1 (e)	5.2 o)
	4.9.2	16.2
Corrective action	4.10.1	N
	4.10.2	N
	4.10.3	N
	4.10.4	N
	4.10.5	16.2
Preventive action	4.11.1	N
	4.11.2	N
Control of records	4.12.1.1	12.1
	4.12.1.2	12.2
	4.12.1.3	12.2
	4.12.1.4	10.7 e)
	4.12.2.1	12.1
	4.12.2.2	N
	4.12.2.3	N
Internal audits	4.13.1	5.3
	4.13.2	5.3
	4.13.3	5.5
	4.13.4	N
Management reviews	4.14.1	5.4
	4.14.2	5.5
Technical requirements General	5.1.1	N
	5.1.2	N
Personnel	5.2.1	6.1
	5.2.2	6.2
	5.2.3	N
	5.2.4	5.2 e)
	5.2.5	6.3
Accommodation and environmental conditions	5.3.1	7.1, 7.2
	5.3.2	7.3
	5.3.3	7.4
	5.3.4	7.5
	5.3.5	7.6
Test and calibration methods and method validation	5.4.1	10.2, 10.1, 10.5
	5.4.2	10.3

Item from contents list of ISO/IEC 17025	*Clause ISO/IEC 17025*	*Clause ISO/IEC Guide25*
	5.4.3	N
	5.4.4	10.4
	5.4.5.1	N
	5.4.5.2	10.4
	5.4.5.3	N
	5.4.6.1	10.2
	5.4.6.2	10.2
	5.4.6.3	N
	5.4.7.1	10.6
	5.4.7.2	10.7
	5.4.7.2 (a)	10.7 b)
	5.4.7.2 (b)	10.7 c)
	5.4.7.2 (c)	10.7 d)
Equipment	5.5.1	8.1
	5.5.2	9.1
	5.5.3	10.1
	5.5.4	N
	5.5.5 (a)	8.4 a)
	5.5.5 (b)	8.4 b)
	5.5.5 (c)	N
	5.5.5 (d)	8.4 d)
	5.5.5 (e)	8.4 f)
	5.5.5 (f)	8.4 g)
	5.5.5 (g)	8.4 h)
	5.5.5 (h)	8.4 i)
	5.5.6	8.2
	5.5.7	8.2
	5.5.8	8.3
	5.5.9	N
	5.5.10	N
	5.5.11	N
	5.5.12	N
Measurement traceability	5.6.1	9.1
	5.6.2.1.1	9.2
	5.6.2.1.2	9.3
	5.6.2.2.1	9.2
	5.6.2.2.2	9.3
	5.6.3.1	9.4, 9.5
	5.6.3.2	9.7
	5.6.3.3	9.6
	5.6.3.4	N

Item from contents list of ISO/IEC 17025	*Clause ISO/IEC 17025*	*Clause ISO/IEC Guide25*
Sampling	5.7.1	10.5
	5.7.2	N
	5.7.3	N
Handling of test and calibration items	5.8.1	11.4
	5.8.2	11.1
	5.8.3	11.2
	5.8.4	11.3
Assuring the quality of test and calibration results	5.9	5.6, 5.6 a)
	5.9 (a)	5.6 c)
	5.9 (b)	5.6 b)
	5.9 (c)	5.6 d)
	5.9 (d)	5.6 e)
	5.9 (e)	5.6 f)
Reporting the results	5.10.1	13.1
	5.10.2. (a)	13.2 a)
	5.10.2. (b)	13.2 b)
	5.10.2. (c)	13.2 c)
	5.10.2. (d)	13.2 d)
	5.10.2 (e)	13.2 h)
	5.10.2. (f)	13.2 e), 13.2f)
	5.10.2. (g)	13.2 g)
	5.10.2. (h)	13.2 i)
	5.10.2. (i)	13.2 k)
	5.10.2. (j)	13.2 m)
	5.10.2 (k)	13.2 n)
	5.10.3.1 (a)	13.2 j)
	5.10.3.1 (b)	N
	5.10.3.1 (c)	13.2 l)
	5.10.3.1 (d)	N
	5.10.3.1 (e)	N
	5.10.3.2 (a)	N
	5.10.3.2 (b)	N
	5.10.3.2 (c)	N
	5.10.3.2 (d)	N
	5.10.3.2 (e)	N
	5.10.3.2 (f)	N
	5.10.4.1 (a)	13.2 j)
	5.10.4.1 (b)	13.2 l)
	5.10.4.1 (c)	N

Item from contents list of ISO/IEC 17025	*Clause ISO/IEC 17025*	*Clause ISO/IEC Guide25*
	5.10.4.2	N
	5.10.4.3	N
	5.10.4.4.	N
	5.10.5	N
	5.10.6	13.3
	5.10.7	13.7
	5.10.8	13.4
	5.10.9	13.5

(N: NOT REFERRED)

Appendix 2

Pre-Laboratory Accreditation Check List

The applicant test or calibration laboratory, who desired to apply to a national accreditation body for granting accreditation and has already prepared for its quality system documentation, should check its quality documentation for its compliance to the requisite requirements of laboratory accreditation standard. The following check list shall be helpful:

A. Application Form check list
B. Quality System Documentation check list

APPLICATION FORM CHECK LIST

The applicant test or calibration laboratory should check the fulfillment of the following requirements in the application form:

1. Whether your laboratory is registered with some statutory body or it is incorporated under relevant act of your country like Indian Partnership Act 1936 or Indian Companies Act 1956?
2. Whether your laboratory's testing or calibration personnel comply to the qualification and experience requirement as stipulated in the respective specific criteria for a particular discipline of testing or calibration?
3. Whether your laboratory has adequate equipment/instrument of appropriate accuracy and capacity?
4. Whether equipments are calibrated and laboratory has certificate of calibration traceable to national or international metrological institution?
5. Whether you have mentioned range and accuracy of test methods in your application form?
6. Whether you have mentioned latest test method specification in your application form?

7. Whether your application has operational organization chart?
8. Whether your laboratory has appointed a quality manager?
9. Have you signed your application?

QUALITY SYSTEM DOCUMENTATION CHECK LIST

The quality system documentation check lists can be divided in the following categories,

(i) Quality Manual check list
(ii) Quality procedures check list
(iii) Standard operating procedures check list

Quality Manual Check List

The Quality Manual check list should cover the individual accreditation element related to quality system or technical competence of the laboratory.

1. Whether Quality Manual describes about ?
   - General information of laboratory
   - Activities of the laboratory
   - Administration of Quality Manual
   - Content list
   - Distribution list
   - Amendment sheet

2. Whether the Quality Manual states about?
   - Status of laboratory (Temporary, Mobile or Permanent)
   - Legal identity of laboratory
   - Nomination of quality manager
   - Technical manager
   - Adequacy of supervisory staff
   - Technical management
   - Integrity and confidentiality
   - Clients' proprietary rights
   - Contractual personnel
   - Interest of conflict
   - Nomination of deputies

3. Whether the Quality Manual describes about?
   - Quality Policy
   - Objective, and
   - Commitment

4. Whether the Quality Manual states about ?
   - Quality system policy
   - Structure of quality system documentation
   - Document control
   - Review of request, tender and contract
   - Sub-contracting of test or calibration
   - Purchase system
   - Client service (client cooperation)
   - Complaint redressel

5. Whether the Quality Manual describes about ?
   - Non-conforming test or calibration work
   - Corrective action
   - Preventive action
   - Record system

6. Whether the Quality Manual has mentioning of
   - Internal audit
   - Internal audit plan
   - Nomination of auditor
   - Carrying out internal audit
   - Corrective action verification
   - Records of internal audit

7. Whether Quality Manual describes about?
   - Management review
   - Management review procedure
   - Follow up action
   - Records

8. Whether the Quality Manual addresses
   - Factors controlling test or calibration reliability
   - Personnel qualification & experience
   - Personnel training plan
   - Personnel training records

9. Whether the Quality Manual describes about ?
   - Accommodation of laboratory
   - Environment control
   - Monitoring of environment controls

- Access to control areas
- Good house keeping

10. Whether the Quality Manual addresses
    - Standard test or calibration method
    - Non-standard validation method
    - Laboratory developed and validated methods
    - Validation records

11. Whether the Quality Manual addresses
    - Uncertainty of measurement
    - Raw data control
    - Raw data record

12. Whether Quality Manual states about records maintained such as equipment log book for
    - Equipment detail
    - Maintenance history
    - Calibration status
    - Calibration programme

13. Whether Quality Manual addresses,
    - Traceability of test or calibration to national/international body

14. Whether the laboratory has reference materials, reference standards or CRM, and traceability is maintained?
15. Whether the laboratory follows sampling before test or calibration of items? Have it addressed in Quality Manual.
16. Whether sample handling is addressed in Quality Manual?
17. Whether the laboratory follows quality assurance for test or calibration and is it addressed in Quality Manual?
18. Whether the test report or calibration report comply to the standard requirement?
19. Whether the Quality Manual has list of quality procedures and their cross reference?
20. Whether the Quality Manual has cross reference for Standard Operating Procedures?
21. Whether the Quality Manual has addressed sub-contracting of test or calibration.
22. Whether Quality Manual states about preventive action for recurring problems and corrective action?

Quality Procedure Check List

The quality system procedures prepared by the laboratory for accreditation elements, related to quality system or technical, for uniformity should follow a check list to ensure,

- Whether standard quality system procedure (QSP) format is followed for every quality system procedure?
- Whether QSP title is mentioned?
- Whether appropriate numbers to QSP and a cross-reference to Quality Manual chapters is maintained?
- Whether responsibility is mentioned in QSP?
- Whether QSP is written in step wise manner?
- Whether QSPs are approved by authorized personnel?
- Whether there is a provision for review of QSP?

Standard Operating Procedures Check List

The Standard Operating Procedures prepared by the laboratory either for maintenance, cleanliness, equipment operation or test or calibration methods should have checklist for their uniformity and correctness. The following may be checked for an appropriate SOP –

- Whether standard format is followed for every Standard Operating Procedures?
- Whether titles of Standard Operating Procedures are mentioned?
- Whether appropriate numbering system for SOPs is followed?
- Whether responsibility is mentioned in SOP?
- Whether equipment range and accuracy are mentioned in SOPs?
- Whether reference to specification, text book or journal is mentioned in SOP?
- Whether SOPs are approved ?
- Whether SOPs have issue date?
- Whether documentation record are maintained for each SOPs?

Quality Records Check List

The laboratory should have a check list for records, which may cover the following,

- Whether records have titles?
- Whether all columns and rows have their respective sub titles?
- Whether records have signature of supervisors or concerned personnel?
- Whether numbering system is followed for record?

Appendix 3

Relevant ISO Guides/ Standards

ISO Guide 2: !991	General terms and their definitions concerning to standardization and related activities
ISO Guide 58:1993	Calibration and testing laboratories accreditation system
ISO Guide 25:1990	General requirement for competence of test or calibration laboratories
ISO Guide 49:1986	Guide for development of Quality Manual for test or calibration laboratories
ISO 9004:1994	Guide lines for quality system documentation
ISO/IEC 17025:1999	General requirements for competence of testing or calibration laboratories
ISO/IEC Guide 43: 1984	Development and operation of laboratory proficiency testing

Appendix 4

Obtaining ISO Publications, Guides or Standards

The following contact points may be accessed for obtaining obtaining ISO publications, guides or standards:

1. http://www.iso.org/iso/en/prods-services/ISOstore/orderinfo.html
2. **CataloguePlus 2004** on CD-ROM has information on all published ISO standards and other publications.
3. **Purchasing from ISO members**

Contact information for Web store, where available

ALBANIE (DPS)
General Directorate of Standardization
"Mine Peza" Str. Nr 143/3
P.O. Box 98
TIRANA

Tel. + 355 42 262 55
Fax + 355 42 471 77
E-mail info@dps.gov.al

ALGERIA (IANOR)
Institut algérien de normalisation
5 et 7 rue Abou Hamou Moussa
(ex-rue Daguerre)
B.P. 104 RP
ALGER

Tel. + 213 21 64 20 75
Fax + 213 21 64 17 61
E-mail ianor@ianor.org
Web www.ianor.org

ANGOLA (IANORQ)
Instituto Angolano de
Normalização e Qualidade
Ministério da Industria
Rua Cerqueira Luikoki N°25, 7° andar
LUANDA

Tel. + 244 2 33 72 94
Fax + 244 2 39 24 00
E-mail ianorq@netangola.com

ARGENTINA (IRAM)
Instituto Argentino de Normalización y
Certificación - IRAM
Perú 552/556
C1068AAB BUENOS AIRES

Tel. + 54 11 43 46 06 02
Fax + 54 11 43 46 06 05
E-mail iram-iso@iram.org.ar
Web www.iram.com.ar

ARMENIA (SARM)
National Institute of Standards and QualityMinistry of Trade and Economic Development
Komitas Avenue 49/2
375051 YEREVAN

Tel. + 374 1 23 70 20
Fax + 374 1 28 56 20
E-mail sarm@sarm.am
Web www.sarm.am

AUSTRALIA (SA)
Standards Australia
286 Sussex Street (corner of Bathurst Street)
SYDNEY, NSW 2000
Postal address/Adresse postale
GPO Box 5420
SYDNEY, NSW 2001

Tel. + 61 2 82 06 60 00
Fax + 61 2 82 06 60 01
E-mail intsect@standards.com.org.au
Web www.standards.org.au/

AUSTRIA (ON)
Österreichisches Normungsinstitut
Austrian Standards Institute
Heinestrasse 38
AT-1020 WIEN

Tel. + 43 1 213 00 610
Fax + 43 1 213 00 609
E-mail iro@on-norm.at
Web www.on-norm.at/

AZERBAÏDJAN (AZSTAND)
State Agency on Standardization, Metrology and
Patents of Azerbaijan Republic
Mardanov Gardashlary str., 124
370078 BAKU

Tel. + 99 412 440 51 54
Fax + 99 412 440 52 24
E-mail smp@azerin.com

BAHRAIN (BSMD)
Directorate of Standards and Metrology
Ministry of Commerce
Building 240, road 1704, block 317
Diplomatic Area
BAHRAIN
Postal address/Adresse postale
Ministry of CommerceP.O. Box 5479
Manama
BAHRAIN

Tel. + 973 17 57 48 71
Fax + 973 17 53 07 30
E-mail bsmd@commerce.gov.bh

BANGLADESH (BSTI)
Bangladesh Standards and Testing Institution
116/A, Tejgaon Industrial Area
DHAKA-1208

Tel. + 88 02 882 14 62
Fax + 88 02 913 15 81
E-mail bsti@bangla.net
Web www.bstibd.org

BARBADOS (BNSI)
Barbados National Standards Institution
Flodden Culloden Road
ST. MICHAEL

Tel. + 1 246 426 38 70
Fax + 1 246 436 14 95
E-mail office@bnsi.com.bb

BELARUS (BELST)
Committee for Standardization,
Metrology and Certification of Belarus
93 Starovilensky Tract
MINSK 220053

Tel. + 375 172 33 52 13
Fax + 375 172 33 25 88
E-mail belgiss-nk@mail.belpak.by
Web www.gosstandart.gov.by

BELGIUM (IBN)
Institut belge de normalisation
Av. de la Brabançonne 29
B-1000 BRUXELLES

Tel. + 32 2 738 01 11
Fax + 32 2 733 42 64
E-mail vanboxstael@ibn.be
Web www.ibn.be

BOLIVIA (IBNORCA)
IInstituto Boliviano de
Normalización y Calidad
Av. Busch N° 1196
(entre calles Honduras y Haití)
Zona Miraflores
Casilla postal N° 5034
LA PAZ

Tel.	+ 591 2 222 37 38
Fax	+ 591 2 222 34 10
E-mail	info@ibnorca.org
Web	www.ibnorca.org

BOSNIA AND HERZEGOVINA (BASMP)
Institute for Standards,
Metrology and Intellectual
Property of Bosnia and Herzegovina
Hamdije emerli a 2
(ENERGOINVEST building)
71000 SARAJEVO

Tel.	+ 387 33 65 27 65
Fax	+ 387 33 65 27 57
E-mail	info@basmp.gov.ba
Web	www.basmp.gov.ba

BOTSWANA (BOBS)
Botswana Bureau of Standards
Plot No. 14391, New Lobatse Road
Gaborone West Industrial
Private Bag BO 48
GABORONE

Tel.	+ 267 31 640 44
Fax	+ 267 31 640 42
E-mail	infoc@hq.bobstandards.bw

BRAZIL (ABNT)
Associação Brasileira de Normas Técnicas
Av. 13 de Maio, n° 13, 28° andar
20003-900 - RIO DE JANEIRO-RJ

Tel.	+ 55 11 37 67 36 18
Fax	+ 55 11 37 67 36 33
E-mail	abnt@abnt.org.br
Web	www.abnt.org.br/

BRUNEI DARUSSALAM (CPRU)
Construction Planning and Research Unit
Ministry of Development
BRUNEI DARUSSALAM

Tel.	+ 673 2 38 10 33
Fax	+ 673 2 38 15 41
E-mail	modcpru@brunet.bn
Web	www.mod.gov.bn

BULGARIA (BDS)
Bulgarian Institute for standardization
21, 6th September Str.
1000 SOFIA

Tel.	+ 359 2 981 00 89
Fax	+ 359 2 980 63 17
E-mail	standards@bds-bg.org
Web	www.bds-bg.org

BURUNDI (BBN)
Bureau burundais de Normalisation et
Contrôle de la Qualité
Boulevard de L'Indépendance, N°21.
BUJUMBURA

Tel.	+ 257 22 18 15
Fax	+ 257 22 55 95
E-mail	bbn@onatel.bi

CANADA (SCC)
Standards Council of Canada
270 Albert Street, Suite 200
OTTAWA, ONTARIO K1P 6N7

Tel.	+ 1 613 238 32 22
Fax	+ 1 613 569 7808
E-mail	info@scc.ca
Web	www.scc.ca

CHILE (INN)
Instituto Nacional de Normalización
Matías Cousiño 64 - 6° piso
Casilla 995 - Correo Central
SANTIAGO

Tel.	+ 56 2 441 03 30
Fax	+ 56 2 445 88 00
E-mail	inn@inn.cl
Web	www.inn.cl

CHINA (SAC)
Standardization Administration of China
4, Zhichun Road
Haidian District
BEIJING 100088

Tel. + 86 10 62 00 06 75
Fax + 86 10 62 03 37 37
E-mail sac@sac.gov.cn
Web www.sac.gov.cn

COLOMBIA (ICONTEC)
Instituto Colombiano de Normas Técnicas y Certificación
Carrera 37 52-95, Edificio ICONTEC
P.O. Box 14237, BOGOTÁ D.C.

Tel. + 57 1 607 88 88
Fax + 57 1 222 14 35
E-mail isocol@icontec.org.co
Web www.icontec.org.co/

CONGO, THE DEMOCRATIC REPUBLIC OF THE (OCC)
Office Congolais de Contrôle
98, Avenue du Port
B.P. 8806
KINSHASA I
Commune de la Gombe

Tel. + 243 880 51 27
Fax + 243 122 19 74
E-mail occ_dir@yahoo.fr

COSTA RICA (INTECO)
Instituto de Normas Técnicas de Costa Rica
Barrio González Flores
Ciudad Científica de la Universidad de Costa Rica
San Pedro de Montes de Oca
SAN JOSÉ
Postal address/Adresse postale
P.O. Box 6189-1000
SAN JOSÉ

Tel. + 506 283 45 22
Fax + 506 283 48 31
E-mail cerodriguez@inteco.or.cr
Web www.inteco.or.cr

COTE D'IVOIRE (CODINORM)
Côte d'Ivoire Normalisation
Angle Rue du Commerce/Bd Botreau Roussel
5e Etage, Immeuble Le Général
Abidjan Plateau
01 BP 1872
ABIDJAN 01

Tel. + 225 20 21 55 12
Fax + 225 20 21 56 11
E-mail codinorm@africaonline.co.ci

CROATIA (DZNM)
State Office for Standardization and Metrology
Ulica grada Vukovara 78
10000 ZAGREB

Tel. + 385 1 610 63 20
Fax + 385 1 610 93 20
E-mail ured.ravnatelja@dznm.hr
Web www.dznm.hr

CUBA (NC)
Oficina Nacional de Normalización (NC)
Calle E No. 261 entre 11 y 13
VEDADO, LA HABANA 10400

Tel. + 53 7 830 00 22
Fax + 53 7 836 80 48
E-mail nc@ncnorma.cu
Web www.nc.cubaindustria.cu

CYPRUS (CYS)
Cyprus Organization for the Promotion of Quality
Ministry of Commerce, Industry and Tourism
NICOSIA 1421

Tel. + 357 22 40 93 06
Fax + 357 22 75 41 03
E-mail gmichaeloudes@cys.mcit.gov.cy

CZECH REPUBLIC (CSNI)
Czech Standards Institute
Biskupský dvur 5
110 02 PRAHA 1

Tel. + 420 2 21 80 21 11
Fax + 420 2 21 80 23 11
E-mail internat.dept@csni.cz
Web www.csni.cz

DENMARK (DS)
Dansk Standard
(Danish Standards Association)
Kollegievej 6
DK-2920 CHARLOTTENLUND

Tel. + 45 39 96 61 01
Fax + 45 39 96 61 02
E-mail dansk.standard@ds.dk
Web www.ds.dk/

ECUADOR (INEN)
Instituto Ecuatoriano de Normalización
Calle Baquerizo Moreno N° E8-29 (454) y Almagro
Edificio INEN
P.O. Box 17-01-3999
QUITO

Tel. + 593 22 56 56 26
Fax + 593 22 56 78 15
E-mail inenfu@andinanet.net
Web www.inen.gov.ec

EGYPT (EOS)
Egyptian Organization for Standardization and Quality Control (EOS)
16 Tadreeb EL-Modarrebeen St.
El-Ameriya
CAIRO

Tel. + 20 2 603 13 49
Fax + 20 2 259 34 80
E-mail moi@idsc.net.eg
Web www.eos.org.eg

EL SALVADOR (CONACYT)
Consejo Nacional de Ciencia y Tecnología
Colonia Médica
Ave. Dr. E. Alvarez y Pasaje
Dr. Guillermo Rodríguez Pacas no. 51
Edificio Espinoza
Apartado postal 3103
SAN SALVADOR

Tel. + 503 226 28 00
Fax + 503 225 62 55
E-mail evanegas@conacyt.gob.sv
Web www.conacyt.gob.sv

ETHIOPIA (QSAE)
Quality and Standards Authority of Ethiopia
P.O. Box 2310
ADDIS ABABA

Tel. + 251 1 46 05 25
Fax + 251 1 46 08 80/81
E-mail qsae@telecom.net.et
Web www.qsae.org

ESTONIA (EVS)
Eesti Standardikeskus
10, Aru Street
10317 Tallinn

Tel. + 372 605 50 50
Fax + 372 605 50 70
E-mail info@evs.ee
Web www.evs.ee

FINLAND (SFS)
Finnish Standards Association SFS
P.O. Box 116
FI-00241 HELSINKI

Tel. + 358 9 149 93 31
Fax + 358 9 146 49 25
E-mail sfs@sfs.fi
Web www.sfs.fi

FRANCE (AFNOR)
Association française de normalisation
11, avenue Francis de Pressensé
F-93571 SAINT DENIS LA PLAINE CEDEX

Tel. + 33 1 41 62 80 00
Fax + 33 1 49 17 90 00
E-mail uari@afnor.fr
Web www.afnor.fr

GERMANY (DIN)
Burggrafenstrasse 6
D-10787 BERLIN
Postal address/Adresse postale
D-10772 BERLIN

Tel. + 49 30 26 01-0
Fax + 49 30 26 01 12 31
E-mail directorate.international@din.de
Web www.din.de

GHANA (GSB)
Ghana Standards Board
P.O. BOX MB 245
ACCRA

Tel. + 233 21 50 14 95
Fax + 233 21 50 00 92
E-mail gsbnep@ghanastandards.org

GREECE (ELOT)
Hellenic Organization for Standardization
313, Acharnon Street
GR- 111 45 ATHENS

Tel. + 30 210 21 20 100
Fax + 30 210 21 20 131
E-mail info@elot.gr
Web www.elot.gr

GUATEMALA (COGUANOR)
Comisión Guatemalteca de Normas
8a. Avenida 10-43, Zona 1, Tercel nivel
GUATEMALA, C.A.

Tel. + 502 2 238 33 31-39 Ext. 3903
Fax + 502 2 238 33 31-39 Ext. 3901
E-mail mbeteta@mail.mineco.gob.gt
Web www.mineco.gob.gt/portal.php

HONG KONG, CHINA (ITCHKSAR)
Innovation and Technology Commission
Quality Services Division Product Standards
Information Bureau
36/F Immigration Tower
7 Gloucester Rd.
Wan Chai
HONG KONG

Tel. + 852 28 29 48 19
Fax + 852 28 24 13 02
E-mail psib@itc.gov.hk
Web www.info.gov.hk/itc

HUNGARY (MSZT)
Magyar Szabványügyi Testület
Üllöi út 25
Pf.24.
H-1450 BUDAPEST 9
PF. 24.

Tel. + 36 1 456 68 00
Fax + 36 1 456 68 23
E-mail isoline@mszt.hu
Web www.mszt.hu

ICELAND (IST)
Icelandic Standards
Laugavegi 178
IS-105 REYKJAVIK
Tel. + 354 520 71 50
Fax + 354 520 71 71
E-mail stadlar@stadlar.is
Web www.stadlar.is

INDIA (BIS)
Bureau of Indian Standards
Manak Bhavan
9 Bahadur Shah Zafar Marg
NEW DELHI 110002

Tel. + 91 11 323 79 91
Fax + 91 11 323 93 99
Telex 316 58 70 bis in
E-mail ird@bis.org.in
Web www.bis.org.in

INDONESIA (BSN)
Badan Standardisasi Nasional
(National Standardization Agency, Indonesia)
Manggala Wanabakti Blok 4, 4th Floor
Jl. Jendral Gatot Subroto
Senayan
JAKARTA 10270

Tel. + 62 21 574 70 43
Fax + 62 21 574 70 45
E-mail bsn@bsn.or.id
Web www.bsn.or.id

IRAN, ISLAMIC REPUBLIC OF (ISIRI)
Institute of Standards and Industrial
Research of Iran
P.O. Box 14155-6139
TEHRAN

Tel. + 98 261 280 60 31-8
Fax + 98 261 280 50 15
E-mail standard@isiri.or.ir
Web www.isiri.org

IRAQ (COSQC)
Central Organization for Standardization &
Quality Control
Council of Ministers
P.O. Box 13032
AL-Jaderiya
BAGHDAD

Tel. + 964 1 778 05 95
Fax + 964 1 718 73 51
E-mail cosqc@uruklink.net

IRELAND (NSAI)
National Standards Authority of Ireland
Glasnevin
DUBLIN-9

Tel.	+ 353 1 807 38 00
Fax	+ 353 1 807 38 38
E-mail	nsai@nsai.ie
Web	www.nsai.ie

ISRAEL (SII)
Standards Institution of Israel
42 Chaim Levanon Street
TEL AVIV 69977

Tel.	+ 972 3 646 51 00
Fax	+ 972 3 641 96 83
E-mail	iso/iec@sii.org.il
Web	www.sii.org.il

ITALY (UNI)
Ente Nazionale Italiano di Unificazione
Via Battistotti Sassi 11/b
I-20133 Milano

Tel.	+ 39 02 70 02 41
Fax	+ 39 02 70 10 61 49
E-mail	uni@uni.com
Web	www.uni.com

JAMAICA (JBS)
Bureau of Standards, Jamaica
6 Winchester Road, P.O. Box 113
KINGSTON 10

Tel.	+ 1 876 926 31 40-5
Fax	+ 1 876 929 47 36
E-mail	info@jbs.org.jm
Web	www.jbs.org.jm

JAPAN (JISC/JSA)
Japanese Industrial Standards Committee
c/o Technical Regulation, Standards and
Conformity Assessment Policy Unit
Ministry of Economy,Trade and Industry
1-3-1, Kasumigaseki, Chiyoda-ku
TOKYO 100 - 8901

Tel.	+ 81 3 35 01 94 71
Fax	+ 81 3 35 80 86 37
E-mail	isojisc@meti.go.jp
Web	www.jisc.go.jp

JORDAN (JISM)
Jordan Institution for Standards and
Metrology, P.O. Box 941287
AMMAN 11194

Tel.	+ 962 6 568 03 16
Fax	+ 962 6 568 10 99
E-mail	jism@nic.net.jo
Web	www.jism.gov.jo

KAZAKHSTAN (KAZMEMST)
Committee for Standardization, Metrology
and Certification
Pushkin str. 166/5
10 Kabanbai batyr Avenue
ASTANA 473000

Tel.	+ 7 317 2 29 90 13
Fax	+ 7 317 2 24 13 03
E-mail	int_rel@memst.kz
Web	www.memst.kz

KENYA (KEBS)
Kenya Bureau of Standards
Kapiti Road, Off Mombasa Road
Behind Belle Vue Cinema
P.O. Box 54974 - 00200, City Square
NAIROBI

Tel.	+ 254 20 60 96 60
Fax	+ 254 20 60 40 31
E-mail	info@kebs.org
Web	www.kebs.org

KOREA, DEMOCRATIC PEOPLE'S REPUBLIC OF (CSK)
Committee for Standardization of the
Democratic
People's Republic of Korea
Inhung 1-Dong, Moranbong District
PYONGYANG

Tel.	+ 85 02 181 11 (ext. 381 89 89)
Fax	+ 85 02 381 44 80
E-mail	saqm@co.chesin.com

KOREA, REPUBLIC OF (KATS)
Korean Agency for Technology and
Standards
Ministry of Commerce, Industry and Energy
2, Joongang-dong, Gwachon-city
KYUNGGI-DO 427-716

Tel. + 82 2 507 68 75
Fax + 82 2 503 79 77
E-mail standard@ats.go.kr
Web www.ats.go.kr

KUWAIT (KOWSMD)
Public Authority for Industry
Standards & Industrial Services Affairs (KOWSMD)
Standards & Metrology Department
Post Box 4690 Safat
KW- 13047 KUWAIT

Tel. + 965 530 26 26
Fax + 965 530 26 25
E-mail kowsmd@pai.gov.kw
Web www.pai.gov.kw

KYRGYZSTAN (NISM)
State Inspection for Standardization and Metrology (KYRGYZST)
197 Panfilova str.
720040 BISHKEK

Tel. + 996 31 2 22 78 84
Fax + 996 31 2 66 13 67
E-mail nism@nism.gov.kg
Web www.nism.gov.kg

LATVIA (LVS)
Latvian Standard
157, Kr. Valdemara Street
RIGA LV-1013

Tel. + 371 7 37 13 08
Fax + 371 7 37 13 24
E-mail lvs@lvs.lv
Web www.lvs.lv

LEBANON (LIBNOR)
Lebanese Standards Institution
Gedco Center 3, Bloc B, 9th floor
Shehab Avenue, between Mekalles & Hayek roundabouts
Sin El Fil - Dekwaneh
BEIRUT
Postal address/Adresse postale
P.O. Box 55120
Sin El Fil
BEIRUT

Tel. + 961 1 48 59 27
Fax + 961 1 48 59 29
E-mail libnor@libnor.org
Web www.libnor.org

LIBYAN ARAB JAMAHIRIYA (LNCSM)
Libyan National Centre for Standardization and Metrology
Industrial Research
Centre Building
P.O. Box 5178
TRIPOLI

Tel. + 218 21 369 30 74
Fax + 218 21 369 30 71
E-mail lncsm90@yahoo.com

LITHUANIA (LST)
Lithuanian Standards Board
T. Kosciuskos g.30
LT-01100 VILNIUS

Tel. + 370 52 70 93 60
Fax + 370 52 2 62 52
E-mail lstboard@lsd.lt
Web www.lsd.lt

LUXEMBOURG (SEE)
Service de l'Energie de l'Etat (SEE)
Organisme Luxembourgeois de Normalisation
34 avenue de la Porte-Neuve
B.P. 10L- 010 LUXEMBOURG

Tel. + 352 46 97 46 1
Fax + 352 46 97 46 39
E-mail see.normalisation@eg.etat.lu
Web www.see.lu

MACAU, CHINA (CPTTM)
Macau Productivity and Technology Transfer Center
Rua de Xangai, 175
Edificio Associação Comercial de Macau 6° andar
MACAU

Tel. + 853 78 13 13
Fax + 853 78 82 33
E-mail cpttm@cpttm.org.mo

MADAGASCAR (BNM)
Bureau de Normes de Madagascar
B.P. 1316
ANTANANARIVO 101

Tel. + 261 202 22 79 70
Fax + 261 202 22 64 26
E-mail bnm@wanadoo.mg

MALAWI (MBS)
Malawi Bureau of Standards
P.O. Box 946
BLANTYRE

Tel. + 265 1 67 04 88
Fax + 265 1 67 07 56
E-mail mbs@malawi.net

MALAYSIA (DSM)
Department of Standards Malaysia (DSM)
Ministry of Science, Technology
and Innovation
Level 1 & 2, Block C4, Parcel C
Federal Government Administrative Centre
62502 PUTRAJAYA

Tel. + 60 3 88 85 80 00
Fax + 60 3 88 88 50 60
E-mail central@dsm.gov.my
Web www.dsm.gov.my

MALTA (MSA)
Malta Standards Authority
Second Floor, Evans Building
Merchants Street
VALLETTA VLT 03

Tel. + 356 21 24 24 20
Fax + 356 21 24 24 06
E-mail info@msa.org.mt
Web www.msa.org.mt

MAURITIUS (MSB)
Mauritius Standards Bureau
Villa Road
MOKA

Tel. + 230 433 36 48
Fax + 230 433 51 50
E-mail msb@intnet.mu
Web msb.intnet.mu

MEXICO (DGN)
Dirección General de Normas
Calle Puente de Tecamachalco N°6
Lomas de Tecamachalco
Sección Fuentes, Naucalpan de Juárez
53950 Mexico

Tel. + 52 5 729 94 80
Fax + 52 5 729 94 84
E-mail iso-mex@economia.gob.mx
Web www.economia.gob.mx

MOLDOVA, REPUBLIC OF (MOLDST)
Department of Standardization and
Metrology
Str. Coca 28
or. CHISINAU 2064

Tel. + 373 22 74 85 88
Fax + 373 22 75 05 81
E-mail moldovastandard@standart.mldnet.com
Web www.standard.md

MONGOLIA (MASM)
Mongolian Agency for Standardization and
Metrology
P.O. Box 48
ULAANBAATAR 210351

Tel. + 976 11 45 83 49
Fax + 976 11 45 80 32
E-mail masm@mongol.net
Web www.mnstandard.com

MOROCCO (SNIMA)
Service de Normalisation Industrielle
Marocaine (SNIMA)
Ministère de l'industrie, du commerce et
de la mise à niveau de l'économie
Angle Avenue Kamal Zebdi et Rue Dadi
Secteur 21 Hay Riad
10100 RABAT

Tel. + 212 37 71 62 14
Fax + 212 37 71 17 98
E-mail snima@mcinet.gov.ma
Web www.mcinet.gov.ma/snima

MOZAMBIQUE (INNOQ)
Instituto Nacional de Normalização e
Qualidade
C.P. 2983
MAPUTO

Tel. + 258 1 30 38 22
Fax + 258 1 30 42 06
E-mail innoq@emilmoz.com

NAMIBIA (NSIQO)
Namibia Standards Information and Quality Office
Ministry of Trade and Industry
Goethe Street, Private Bag 13340
WINDHOEK

Tel. + 264 61 283 71 11
Fax + 264 61 22 02 27
E-mail ndishishi@mti.gov.na

NEPAL (NBSM)
Nepal Bureau of Standards and Metrology (NBSM)
P.O. Box 985
Sundhara
KATHMANDU

Tel. + 977 1 435 06 89
Fax + 977 1 435 06 89
Telegram gunis
E-mail nbsm@nbsm.gov.np

NETHERLANDS (NEN)
Nederlands Normalisatie-instituut
Vlinderweg 6
NL-2623 AX DELFT
Postal address/Adresse postale
P.O. Box 5059
NL-2600 GB DELFT

Tel. + 31 15 2 69 03 90
Fax + 31 15 2 69 01 90
E-mail info@nen.nl
Web www.nen.nl

NEW ZEALAND (SNZ)
Standards New Zealand
Radio New Zealand House
155 The Terrace
WELLINGTON 6001
Postal address/Adresse postale
Private Bag 2439
WELLINGTON 6020
Tel. + 64 4 498 59 90
Fax + 64 4 498 59 94
E-mail snz@standards.co.nz
Web www.standards.co.nz

NICARAGUA (DTNM)
Dirección de Tecnología, Normalización y Metrología
Ministerio de Fomento, Industria y Comercio
Apartado postal No. 8
MANAGUA

Tel. + 505 267 01 61 Ext. 1032
Fax + 505 267 20 19
E-mail dtnm@mific.gob.ni
Web www.mific.gob.ni

NIGER (DNQM)
Direction de la Normalisation, de la Qualité et de la Métrologie
Ministère du Commerce, de l'Industrie, de l'Artisanat et de la Promotion du Secteur privé
Boîte postale 480
NIAMEY
Tel. + 227 73 69 50
Fax + 227 73 21 50
E-mail dnqm2002@yahoo.fr

NIGERIA (SON)
Standards Organisation of Nigeria
Plot 13/14 Victoria Arobieke St.
Lekki Peninsula Scheme 1
LAGOS

Tel. + 234 1 27 08 247
Fax + 234 1 27 08 246
E-mail info@sononline-ng.org
Web www.sononline-ng.org

NORWAY (SN)
Standards Norway
Strandveien 18LYSAKER
PO Box 242
1366 LYSAKER

Tel. + 47 67 83 86 00
Fax + 47 67 83 86 01
E-mail info@standard.no
Web www.standard.no

OMAN (DGSM)
Directorate General for Specifications and Measurements
Ministry of Commerce and Industry
P.O. Box 550 - Postal code No. 113
MUSCAT

Tel. + 968 771 32 38
Fax + 968 771 59 92
E-mail dgsm123@omantel.net.om
Web www.mocioman.org

PAKISTAN (PSQCA)
Pakistan Standards and Quality Control Authority
Block #77, Pakistan Secretariat
KARACHI-74400

Tel +92 21 920 62 61
Fax +92 21 920 62 63
E-mail psqcadg@super.net.pk
Web www.psqca.com.pk

PANAMA (COPANIT)
Comisión Panameña de Normas Industriales y Técnicas
Edificio Plaza Edison, Tercer Piso
Avenida Ricardo J. Alfaro y Calle El Paical
Apartado 9658
PANAMA 4

Tel. + 507 360 06 00 Ext. 2388 to 2394
Fax + 507 360 07 21
E-mail dgnti@mici.gob.pa
Web www.mici.gob.pa

PAPUA NEW GUINEA (NISIT)
National Institute of Standards and Industrial Technology
P.O. Box 3042
BOROKO
National Capital District

Tel. + 675 323 18 52
Fax + 675 325 87 93
E-mail pngnisit@nisit.gov.pg
Web www.nisit.gov.pg

PARAGUAY (INTN)
Instituto Nacional de Tecnología y Normalización (INTN)
Av. Artigas 3973
Casilla de Correo 967
ASUNCIÓN

Tel. + 595 21 29 01 60
Fax + 595 21 29 08 73
E-mail intn@intn.gov.py

PERU (INDECOPI)
Instituto Nacional de Defensa de la Competencia y de la Protección de la Propiedad Intelectual
Calle La Prosa 138
San Borja
LIMA 41

Tel. + 51 1 224 78 00
Fax + 51 1 224 03 48
E-mail farrunategui@indecopi.gob.pe
Web www.indecopi.gob.pe

PHILIPPINES (BPS)
Bureau of Product Standards
Department of Trade and Industry
3rd Floor Trade and Industry Building
361 Sen. Gil J. Puyat Avenue
Makati City
METRO MANILA 1200

Tel. + 63 2 751 31 23
Fax + 63 2 890 48 52
E-mail bps@dti.dti.gov.ph
Web www.bps.dti.gov.ph

POLAND (PKN)
Polish Committee for Standardizationul.
Swietokrzyska 14
P.O. Box 411PL-00-050 WARSZAWA

Tel. + 48 22 556 75 91
Fax + 48 22 556 77 86
E-mail pl.isonb@pkn.pl
Web www.pkn.pl

PORTUGAL (IPQ)
Instituto Português da Qualidade
Rua António Gião, 2
P-2829-513 CAPARICA

Tel. + 351 21 294 81 00
Fax + 351 21 294 81 01
E-mail ipq@mail.ipq.pt
Web www.ipq.pt

QATAR (QS)
Qatar General Organization for Standards and Metrology
Ministry of Finance, Economy and Commerce
P.O. Box 23277DOHA

Tel. + 974 447 98 05
Fax + 974 447 90 52
E-mail standard@qatar.net.qa

ROMANIA (ASRO)
Asociatia de Standardizare din Romania
Str. Mendeleev 21-25, 010362
Sector 1, BUCURESTI

Tel. + 40 1 211 32 96
Fax + 40 1 210 08 33
E-mail international@asro.ro
Web www.asro.ro

RUSSIAN FEDERATION (GOST R)
Federal Agency on Technical Regulating and Metrology
Leninsky Prospekt 9
MOSCOW, V-49, GSP-1, 119991

Tel. + 7 095 236 40 44
Fax + 7 095 236 62 31
E-mail info@gost.ru
Web www.gost.ru

RWANDA (RBS)
Rwanda Bureau of Standards
P.O. Box 7099
KIGALI

Tel. + 250 58 29 45
Fax + 250 58 33 05
E-mail orn@rwanda1.com

SAINT LUCIA (SLBS)
Saint Lucia Bureau of Standards
Bisee Industrial Estate
CP 5412
CASTRIES

Tel. + 1 758 453 00 49
Fax + 1 758 452 35 61
E-mail slbs@candw.lc
Web www.slbs.org.lc

SAUDI ARABIA (SASO)
Saudi Arabian Standards Organization
Imam Saud Bin Abdul Aziz Bin Mohammed Road (West End)
P.O. Box 3437
RIYADH 11471

Tel. + 966 1 452 00 00
Fax + 966 1 452 00 86
E-mail saso@saso.org.sa
Web www.saso.org.sa

SENEGAL (ASN)
Ministère de l'Industrie et de l'Artisanat
122 bis avenue André Peytavin
Boîte postale 4037
DAKAR

Tel. + 221 827 64 01
Fax + 221 827 64 12
E-mail asnor@sentoo.sn

SERBIA AND MONTENEGRO (ISSM)
Institution for tandardization of Serbian and Montenegro
Stevana Brakusa 2
Post. fah 2105
11030 BELGRADE

Tel. + 381 11 54 70 96
Fax + 381 11 35 41 258
E-mail jus@jus.org.yu
Web www.jus.org.yu

SEYCHELLES (SBS)
Seychelles Bureau of Standards
Pointe Larue
MAHÉ
Postal address/Adresse postale
P.O. Box 953
Victoria
MAHÉ

Tel. + 248 38 04 00
Fax + 248 37 51 51
E-mail sbsorg@seychelles.net
Web www.seychelles.net/sbsorg

SINGAPORE (SPRING SG)
Standards, Productivity and Innovation Board
2 Bukit Merah Central
SINGAPORE 159835

Tel. + 65 62 79 18 05
Fax + 65 62 78 69 90
E-mail stn@spring.gov.sg
Web www.spring.gov.sg

SLOVAKIA (SUTN)
Slovak Standards Institute
P.O.Box 246, Karloveská 63
SK-840 00 BRATISLAVA 4

Tel. + 421 2 60 29 44 74
Fax + 421 2 65 41 18 88
E-mail ms_post@sutn.gov.sk
Web www.sutn.gov.sk

SLOVENIA (SIST)
Slovenian Institute for Standardization
Smartinska 140
SI-1000 LJUBLJANA

Tel. + 386 1 478 30 13
Fax + 386 1 478 30 94
E-mail sist@sist.si
Web www.sist.si

SOUTH AFRICA (SABS)
South African Bureau of Standards
1 Dr Lategan Rd, Groenkloof
Private Bag X191
PRETORIA 0001

Tel. + 27 12 428 79 11
Fax + 27 12 344 15 68
E-mail info@sabs.co.za
Web www.sabs.co.za

SPAIN (AENOR)
Asociación Española de Normalización y Certificación, Génova, 6
E- 28004 MADRID

Tel. + 34 91 432 60 00
Fax + 34 91 310 49 76
E-mail aenor@aenor.es
Web www.aenor.es

SRI LANKA (SLSI)
Sri Lanka Standards Institution
17 Victoria Place
Off Elvitigala Mawatha
P.O. Box 17
COLOMBO 08

Tel. + 94 11 67 15 74
Fax + 94 11 67 15 79
E-mail dgslsi@sltnet.lk
Web www.nsf.ac.lk/slsi

SUDAN (SSMO)
Sudanese Standards and Metrology Organization
P.O. Box 13573
KHARTOUM

Tel. + 249 183 77 74 80
Fax + 249 183 79 80 11
E-mail ssmo@sudanmail.net

SWAZILAND (SQAS)
Standardization and Quality Assurance Section
Ministry of Enterprise and Employment
P.O. Box 451
MBABANE

Tel. + 268 404 75 09/10
Fax + 268 404 30 55
E-mail mee@realnet.co.sz

SWEDEN (SIS)
SIS, Swedish Standards Institute
Sankt Paulsgatan 6
STOCKHOLM
Postal address/Adresse postale
SE-118 80 STOCKHOLM

Tel. + 46 8 55 55 20 00
Fax + 46 8 55 55 20 01
E-mail info@sis.se
Web www.sis.se

SWITZERLAND (SNV)
Swiss Association for Standardization
Bürglistrasse 29
CH-8400 Winterthur

Tel. + 41 52 224 54 54
Fax + 41 52 224 54 74
E-mail info@snv.ch
Web www.snv.ch

SYRIAN ARAB REPUBLIC (SASMO)
Syrian Arab Organization for Standardization and Metrology
P.O. Box 11836
DAMASCUS

Tel.	+ 963 11 452 98 23
Fax	+ 963 11 452 82 14
E-mail	sasmo@net.sy
Web	www.sasmo.org

TANZANIA, UNITED REPUBLIC OF (TBS)
Tanzania Bureau of StandardsUbungo Area
Morogoro Road/Sam Nujoma Road
DAR ES SALAAM
Postal address/Adresse postale
P.O. Box 9524
DAR ES SALAAM

Tel.	+ 255 22 245 02 98
Fax	+ 255 22 245 09 59
E-mail	info@tbs.or.tz
Web	www.tbs-tz.org

THAILAND (TISI)
Thai Industrial Standards Institute
Ministry of Industry
Rama VI Street
BANGKOK 10400

Tel.	+ 66 2 202 34 00-2
Fax	+ 66 2 354 30 41
E-mail	intrelat@tisi.go.th
Web	www.tisi.go.th

THE FORMER YUGOSLAV REPUBLIC OF MACEDONIA (ISMR)
"Standardization Institute of the Republic of Macedonia"
Ministry of Economy
Vasil Glavinov bb, blok 10 - mezanin
1000 SKOPJE

Tel.	+ 389 2 329 89 44
Fax	+ 389 2 329 89 45
E-mail	ezov.mihail@zsm.gov.mk

TRINIDAD AND TOBAGO (TTBS)
Trinidad and Tobago Bureau of Standards1-2
Century Drive Trincity Industrial Estate
TUNAPUNA
Postal address/Adresse postale
P.O. Box 467
PORT OF SPAIN

Tel.	+ 1 868 662 88 27
Fax	+ 1 868 663 43 35
E-mail	ttbs@ttbs.org.tt
Web	www.ttbs.org.tt

TUNISIA (INORPI)
Institut National de la Normalisation et de la Propriété Industrielle
Rue 8451 n°8 par la rue Alain Savary BP 57
Cité El Khadra
1003 TUNIS

Tel.	+ 216 71 78 59 22
Fax	+ 216 71 78 15 63
E-mail	INORPI@email.ati.tn
Web	www.inorpi.ind.tn

TURKEY (TSE)
Türk Standardlari Enstitüsü
Necatibey Cad. 112
Bakanliklar
TR-06100 ANKARA

Tel.	+ 90 312 417 83 30
Fax	+ 90 312 425 43 99
E-mail	usm@tse.org.tr
Web	www.tse.org.tr

TURKMENISTAN (MSIT)
Major State Service "Turkmenstandartlary"
Seydi, 14
744000 ASHGABAT

Tel.	+ 993 1 251 14 94
Fax	+ 993 1 251 04 98
E-mail	nmsit@online.tm

UGANDA (UNBS)
Uganda National Bureau of Standards
P.O. Box 6329
KAMPALA

Tel.	+ 256 41 22 23 67
Fax	+ 256 41 28 61 23
E-mail	unbs@afsat.com
Web	www.unbs.org

UKRAINE (DSSU)
State Committee on Technical Regulation and Consumer Policy of Ukraine
(Derzhspozhivstandard of Ukraine)
174, Gorkiy Street, GSP 03680
KYIV-150

Tel.	+ 380 44 226 29 71
Fax	+ 380 44 226 29 70
E-mail	dstu@dssu.gov.ua
Web	www.dssu.gov.ua

UNITED ARAB EMIRATES (ESMA)
Emirates Authority for Standardization and Metrology
P.O. Box 2166
ABU DHABI

Tel.	+ 971 2 671 11 10
Fax	+ 971 2 671 59 99
E-mail	esma@uae.gov.ae

UNITED KINGDOM (BSI)
British Standards Institution
389 Chiswick High Road
GB-LONDON W4 4AL

Tel.	+ 44 208 996 90 00
Fax	+ 44 208 996 74 00
E-mail	standards.international@bsi-global.com
Web	www.bsi-global.com

URUGUAY (UNIT)
Instituto Uruguayo de Normas Técnicas
Pza. Independencia 812, Piso 2
MONTEVIDEO

Tel.	+ 598 2 901 20 48
Fax	+ 598 2 902 16 81
E-mail	unit-iso@unit.org.uy
Web	www.unit.org.uy

USA (ANSI)
American National Standards Institute
1819 L Street, NW
WASHINGTON, DC 20036
Postal address/Adresse postale
25 West 43rd Street, Fourth Floor
NEW YORK, N.Y. 10036

Tel.	+ 1 212 642 49 00
Fax	+ 1 212 398 00 23
E-mail	info@ansi.org
Web	www.ansi.org

UZBEKISTAN (UZSTANDARD)
Agency for Standardization, Metrology and Certification of Uzbekistan
Ulitsa Faroby st., 333 "A"
700049 TACHKENT

Tel.	+ 998 71 144 96 01
Fax	+ 998 71 114 37 81
E-mail	uzst@standart.uz
Web	www.standart.uz

VENEZUELA (FONDONORMA)
Fondo para la Normalización y Certificación de la Calidad
Avenida Andrés Bello
Edf. Torre Fondo Común, Pisos 11 y 12
Apartado Postal 51116
Sabana Grande
CARACAS 1050-A

Tel.	+ 58 212 575 41 11
Fax	+ 58 212 574 13 12
E-mail	central@fondonorma.org.ve
Web	www.fondonorma.org.ve

VIET NAM (TCVN)
Directorate for Standards and Quality
Hoang Quoc Viet Street
HANOI

Tel.	+ 84 4 791 16 33
Fax	+ 84 4 791 15 95
E-mail	qhqt1@hn.vnn.vn
Web	http://tcvn.gov.vn

YEMEN (YSMO)
Yemen Standardization, Metrology & Quality Control Organization
AL-Zoberi Street
Industrial Complex
SANA'A

Tel.	+ 967 1 40 86 08/9
Fax	+ 967 1 40 26 36
E-mail	YSMQCO@y.net.ye

ZIMBABWE (SAZ)
Standards Association of Zimbabwe
Northend Close
Northridge Park
Borrowdale
HARARE
Postal address/Adresse postale
P.O. Box 2259
HARARE

Tel.	+ 263 4 88 20 17/8/9
Fax	+ 263 4 88 20 20
E-mail	info@saz.org.zw

Reader's Notes

Reader's Notes

Reader's Notes